CHAIR YOGA

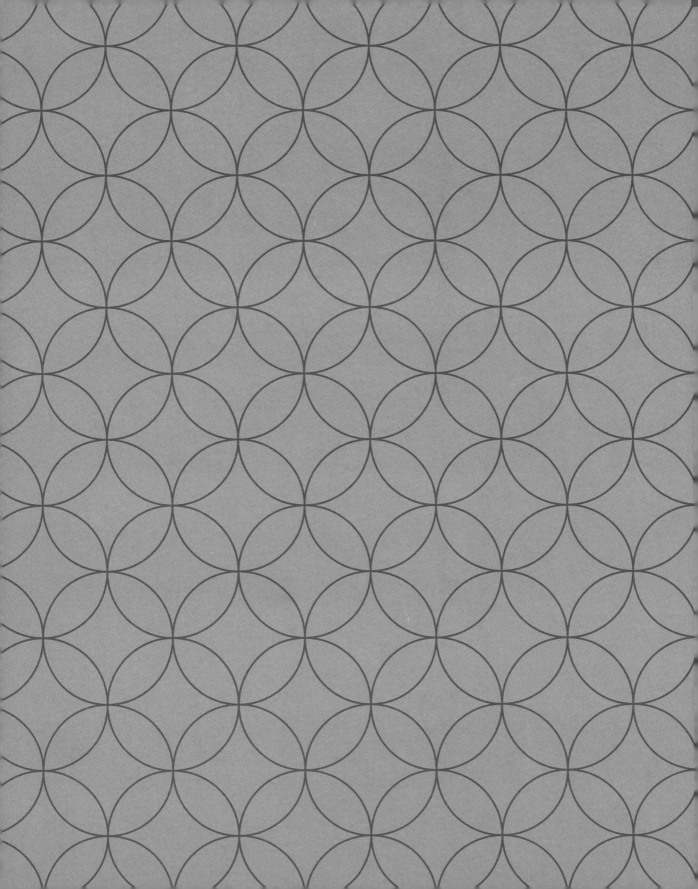

CHAIR YOGA

Accessible Sequences to Build
Strength, Flexibility, and Inner Calm

Christina D'Arrigo
Illustrated by Christy Ni

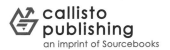
callisto
publishing
an imprint of Sourcebooks

Copyright © 2021 by Callisto Publishing LLC
Cover and internal design © 2021 by Callisto Publishing LLC
Illustrations © Christy Ni, 2021. Author photograph courtesy of Allison Armfield.
Interior and Cover Designer: Jill Lee
Art Producer: Tom Hood
Editor: Eun H. Jeong
Production Editor: Jenna Dutton
Production Manager: Riley Hoffman

Callisto and the colophon are registered trademarks of Callisto Publishing LLC.

Published by Callisto Publishing LLC C/O Sourcebooks LLC
P.O. Box 4410, Naperville, Illinois 60567-4410
(630) 961-3900
callistopublishing.com

Printed and bound in China
OGP 2

I would like to dedicate
this book to my grandparents—
they mean so much to me,
and I know how much they love
their chair yoga and
exercise classes.

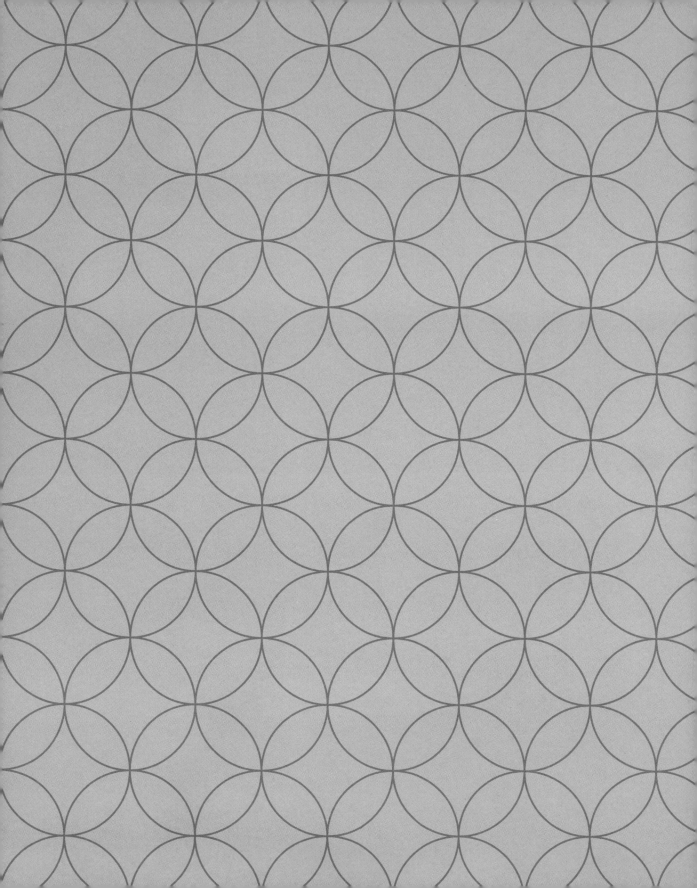

CONTENTS

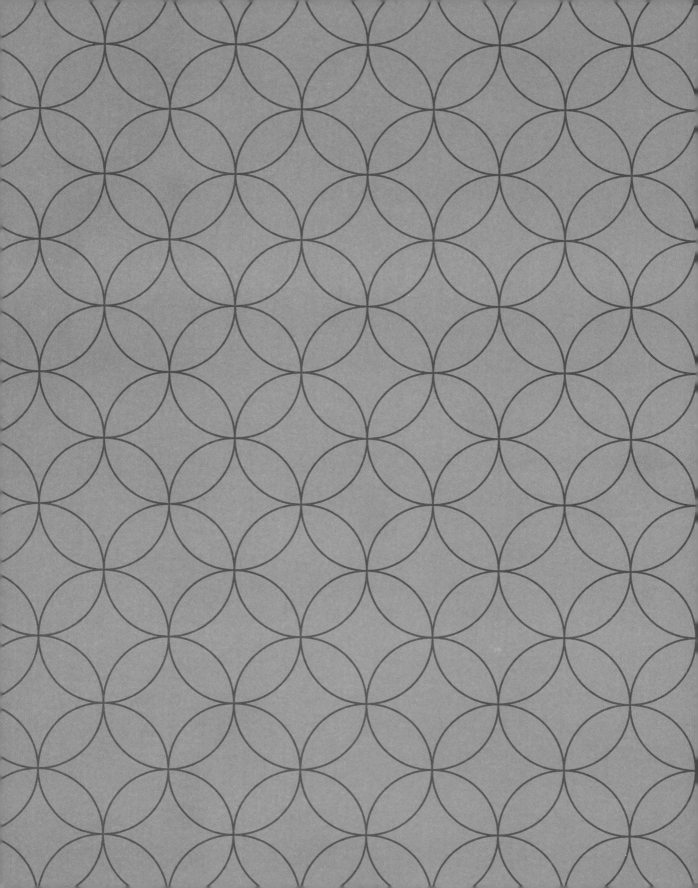

INTRODUCTION

HELLO, I'm Christina! I've been practicing yoga since 2008 and have been teaching it since 2014. I have also completed more than 500 hours of yoga teacher training. I'm a published author and I teach yoga online to tens of thousands of people from all over the world on my YouTube channel, Yoga with Christina. I feel very fortunate to have the opportunity to help many people across the globe find peace, healing, and strength throughout all levels and stages of their yoga journey.

This book will help you discover a new way to practice yoga that you may not have even known was possible: in a chair. Adding a chair to your practice can provide a new level of ease, comfort, mobility, and stability that isn't available in other forms of yoga. Chair yoga is a great way to build strength, gain flexibility, and add more relaxation into your life in a simple and accessible way. You'll likely feel more in control of your health than ever. It helps you maintain a healthy mind and body, and even enhances your overall wellness if you practice it with patience and make time for it in your daily routine.

Chair yoga makes yoga practice safe and accessible for all types of people. You may have picked up this book because you're recovering from an injury or surgery, or perhaps you have certain physical restrictions due to pregnancy, a health condition, age, or available space. This book will be a great resource for you. You can take comfort knowing that you won't be twisting into any uncomfortable or confusing positions. The poses and sequences in this book are gentle, simple, and easy to follow. The routines are customizable to suit your needs and your schedule, and you are in full control of what you choose to practice. You can start and stop anytime you like; practicing for even a few minutes a day can make a significant difference in your life. Just remember to have patience and be kind to yourself along the way. I really hope you enjoy this book and all that it has to offer.

HOW TO USE THIS BOOK

This book is designed to meet your current needs through four sequences: Warm Up, Begin Gently, Tone and Flow, and Unwind and Sleep. You can use these sequences to slowly and gently work your way up to a more challenging yoga practice, or to add relaxation and increase mobility throughout your whole body. The four sequences offer a range of different poses at varying levels, and you can use the sequences as a complete program or pick and choose which poses are right for you in any particular moment. I provide 10-minute and 20-minute programs for each sequence after the warm-up so you can follow each as your schedule allows.

Warm Up: You can begin each practice with this simple warm-up sequence to help prepare your body to move more easily.

Begin Gently: Designed for beginners and those with injuries or restrictions, this sequence offers poses that you can do simply seated in the chair.

Tone and Flow: The poses in this sequence are slightly more dynamic and incorporate standing to provide you with some gentle ways to build strength, stamina, and flexibility.

Unwind and Sleep: Use this sequence for cooling and calming down the body after longer practice sessions, or use it on its own as a way to relax the mind and body.

For each pose, I offer tips on variations you can use to make your practice as comfortable, safe, and fulfilling as possible, while also accommodating any physical limitations you might experience. I'll also highlight the health benefits of each pose and how you can incorporate them into your practice, as well as any cautions you'll need to take.

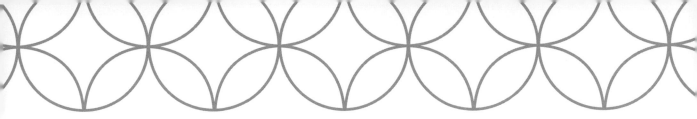

WHO SHOULD USE THIS BOOK

Whether you're a complete yoga beginner or more experienced practitioner, this book can help you practice new poses or extend your range of motion. It's also a great choice if you're a senior or recovering from an injury, surgery, or giving birth—anything where you're dealing with decreased mobility or certain conditions that restrict your movement and stamina. You'll also enjoy this book if you often have to remain seated for long periods at work or on long-haul flights.

The sequences and suggestions in this book are beneficial for all ages and levels of yoga experience. They're designed to be accessible to people with a wide range of physical injuries and restrictions. If you struggle with balance, mobility, and stamina, these routines are especially meant for you. Adding a chair to your practice makes it possible to experience the benefits of yoga in your life while still being kind and gentle to your body.

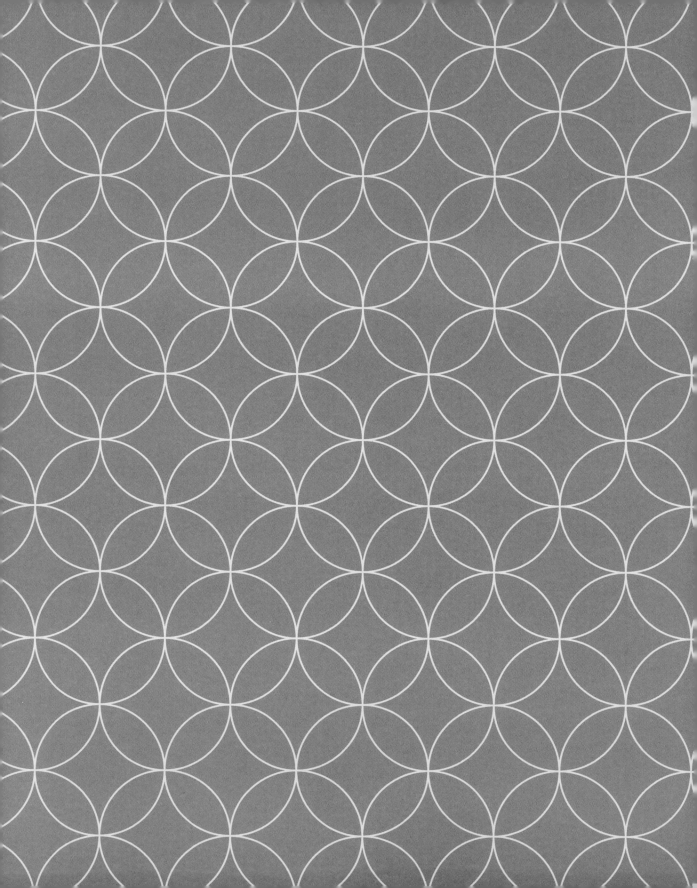

GET STARTED WITH CHAIR YOGA

In this chapter, you'll learn about how and why this particular type of yoga is so helpful for people who face physical and mobility challenges. I'll share the benefits of bringing chair yoga into your life and how you can practice it in a way that is gentle and easily accessible.

I'll also go into detail about how to set up your physical space, your body, and your mind to get the most out of chair yoga. With these tips and suggestions, you'll be able to start your practice in an easy and comfortable way.

Why Chair Yoga?

There are many benefits of yoga, such as increasing flexibility, building strength, reducing anxiety, and improving lung function. But it can often be quite challenging or even intimidating for certain groups of people who worry that their bodies aren't up to the task. In these cases, adding a chair to your yoga practice can be extremely helpful. It will allow you to reap the benefits of yoga that may have previously been out of reach.

Chair yoga can be especially helpful for people who have conditions—such as multiple sclerosis or arthritis—that limit mobility. For those with health issues and movement restrictions, adding a chair can eliminate the need to support the full weight of your body. You can still get the benefits of moving your joints and stretching your muscles without the extra effort of supporting your body weight. This often provides relief for stiff muscles and can make it easier to move and mobilize the joints during everyday life.

If you have an injury in your hands, wrists, knees, ankles, shoulders, or neck, the chair can help you keep the injured area stable while you move and work the rest of your body. Injuries often cause people to lose their stamina, strength, and flexibility throughout their body, but chair yoga helps keep muscles and joints active and healthy by providing stability and support.

It can also benefit people who have trouble reaching up and folding forward, bending and straightening their limbs, or with overall joint mobility. Using a chair when practicing yoga can provide support and stability for those who may be experiencing issues with the functionality of the balance organ in the inner ear, which can cause feelings of being off-balance. This imbalance can increase the risk of falling over and potentially injuring the body, which makes typical yoga asanas (the physical aspect of yoga) more dangerous. Chair yoga can make the whole process feel much safer, more comfortable, and easily attainable.

But chair yoga isn't just for people with injuries or mobility issues. It can also help those whose jobs require them to sit at a desk for eight hours or more, or people who regularly take long-haul flights. Sitting in a chair while practicing *pranayama* (yogic breathing exercises) and meditation can be beneficial for everyone (see page 126 for yogic breathwork). Even just placing your feet flat on the floor can help with feeling calmer and more grounded.

Once you learn and understand the basic movements in a chair yoga practice and feel comfortable with the poses and sequences, you can later expand upon them to set yourself up for a well-rounded and greatly beneficial yoga practice.

Mobility vs. Flexibility

Flexibility and mobility are two words you might hear often in relation to yoga, but what is the difference, exactly? Put simply, flexibility relates to the range of motion in muscles and how far they lengthen. Mobility, on the other hand, relates to a joint's ability to move actively and efficiently. So although you might be flexible in certain areas of your body, you still may not be able to complete certain movements without feeling restricted. A healthy form of flexibility and mobility in the body requires muscle strength and stability. Fortunately, chair yoga can help you improve both.

Prepare for the Practice

There are some simple tips that will make your chair yoga practice easier and more comfortable. These suggestions will not only make the physical practice more enjoyable, but they'll also help you get the most out of your yoga practice so you can feel great before, during, and afterward.

Dress for Yoga

To make sure that you're not physically restricted in any way, wear comfortable clothing while practicing yoga. You can wear anything that allows you to readily move your limbs and bend forward without restriction.

Gather Your Supplies

You'll need a sturdy, solid, and armless chair that will remain in one place as you move. You can also place a yoga mat under the chair to prevent slippage. It's a good idea to have a bottle of water nearby for after your practice. You may also find it helpful to have a yoga strap (or a strap substitute, such as a belt or scarf), or any other yoga props specified in the instructions, such as blankets, blocks, or a bolster. You can use books as a substitute for the block and large, sturdy pillows as a substitute for a bolster.

Blocks and bolsters help support your body in certain poses where the full expression of the pose is not possible due to physical limitations or injury. For instance, if you cannot bend down and place your hands flat on the floor, you can place yoga blocks under your hands to essentially raise the floor up to meet your comfort level of bending and flexibility. Bolsters do the same thing, but are a bit softer, so they are better for sitting on top of to alleviate pressure in the joints when sitting down.

Be Mindful of Your Breath

In yoga, all breathing—both inhales and exhales—typically occurs through the nose. So as a general rule throughout this book, breathe in and out through your nose unless otherwise specified.

It may be overwhelming when you're first starting out with your practice, which might cause you to hold your breath due to concentration. But it's important that you breathe deeply as you're moving and follow the breath cues in the instructions to make sure you're getting the most out of your practice.

Observe How You Feel Before and After

Take a moment before and after your yoga practice to notice how you are feeling in both your body and your mind. This will help you understand whether the practice may be too challenging or too easy for you, and will help you gauge how to proceed the next time you practice.

Make It Your Own

Beginning a chair yoga practice should be an enjoyable and relaxing experience. You can begin at your own pace, take things slowly, and choose which movements are right for you. Don't put any pressure on yourself to get things right or perfect. As long as the movement feels good in your body, that's all that matters.

Each body is different, and your poses will likely look different from the illustrations or anyone else you may be practicing with. It's also perfectly fine if your body has changed and movements feel different to you now from how they may have felt in the past. Be realistic about your limitations and pay attention to your body's signals and cues. Be understanding and kind to yourself while you are practicing. It's very important not to force your body to do something it's not ready for.

If at any point during your practice you feel shortness of breath or dizziness, stop the movement, sit upright, and breathe deeply through your nose. Also, if you ever feel any pain in your joints (any part of your body where two bones are fitted together) while doing a particular movement, stop doing that movement and begin the next one in the sequence if you're feeling well enough to do so.

It's important to have compassion for yourself and your body, and to treat yourself with kindness and patience. Never force yourself into a movement. Instead, have faith that practicing regularly will help you eventually achieve more with your body, but it should be a slow and consistent process. Take your time and focus on what is best for you. Even practicing yoga for just a few minutes a day will help you see improvements in your health and overall wellbeing.

The Story of Yoga

Did you know that yoga is far more than just exercise? In fact, the physical poses that we now know as "yoga" are only one component of a much larger series of physical, spiritual, and mental disciplines that yoga has to offer. Yoga is an ancient and sacred practice that originated in India and dates back to about 3000 BCE. The asanas, or physical postures, in yoga were created as a way to make the body more limber and able to maintain a still, seated position for long periods of time in meditation. The main purpose of a well-rounded yoga practice was originally to achieve spiritual growth through meditation and guidelines of how to go about your everyday life.

There are many physical benefits to practicing yoga on a regular basis. Even if you're able to practice only once a week or once every couple of weeks, over time you'll definitely begin to notice a difference. Some of the benefits include increased flexibility and mobility in your muscles and joints, increased strength, improved stamina, improved cardiovascular health, injury recovery and prevention, and improvement in your overall energy levels.

There are also many emotional benefits to having a regular yoga practice. With the physical postures of yoga, you will increase endorphins and other hormones in your body such as dopamine and adrenaline. These are chemicals produced by your body that help you feel more positive, happy, and less stressed.

Along with helping you feel more positive, yoga and meditation can also add more mental clarity. By adding meditation to your physical yoga practice, you will begin to understand yourself on a different level and be able to handle the stresses of daily life in a whole new way. Even just by meditating for several minutes each day, you'll eventually notice a huge difference.

It's important to understand which areas of your health you would like to work on, and then compose a yoga practice that would most benefit those areas according to your personal needs. Everyone's body is different and everyone is on their own path, so yoga may provide you with benefits in a different way than it does for your neighbor. For instance, the person practicing next to you may have gone through a physical transformation after practicing yoga for several months, while you may have significantly improved your strength and stamina.

Having a regular yoga practice is beneficial on so many levels and in many different ways. You are on your own journey and the only way to find out how yoga will benefit you is to begin your personal practice and gradually understand what yoga can do for you and your life.

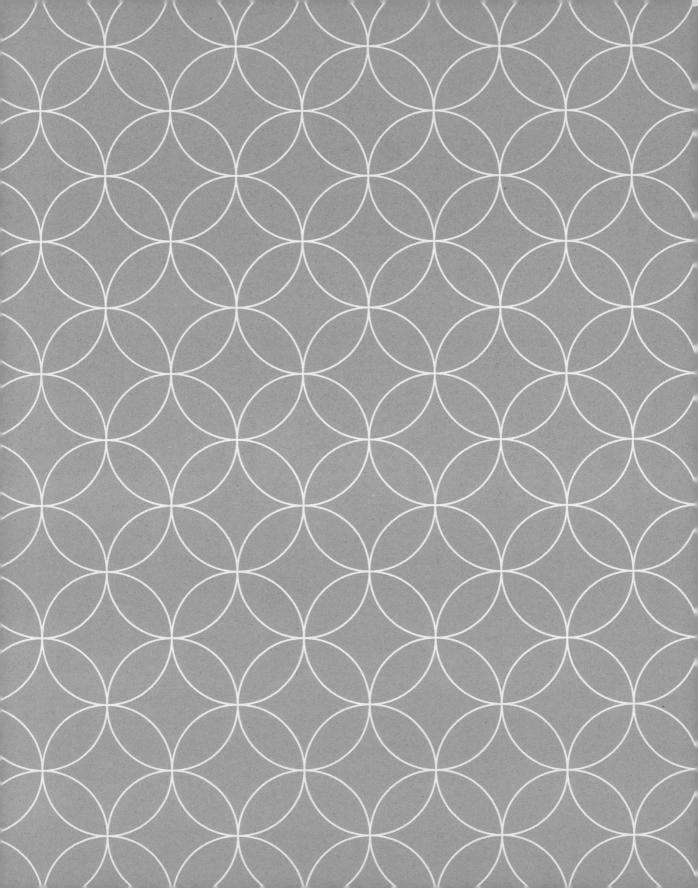

WARM UP

In this chapter, I'll share a short and gentle warm-up chair yoga routine. Beginning each of your chair yoga sessions with this routine will help lubricate your joints, warm up your muscles, release any stiffness, and generally help you feel ready to move. You'll stay in a seated position the entire time, so it's a nice, gentle way to get the body moving before you begin the other sequences.

You can also use this as a stand-alone sequence if you're short on time or if you'd like to keep your practice simple for now. Perhaps you are still recovering from an injury or you are gently working your way up to building more stamina. This would be a great short and simple chair yoga routine to start with.

Chair Mountain Pose (Chair Tadasana)

Body Areas Utilized: Back muscles, front of the chest, shoulders

Good For: Calming the body and mind, feeling more grounded

Instructions

1. Sit on the chair, leaving a bit of space behind you.

2. Lengthen your spine and reach, simultaneously exerting your energy up through the top of your head and down through your sits bones into the seat of the chair.

3. Place your feet flat on the ground at hip-distance apart and keep your legs parallel.

4. Put your palms face-down on top of your upper thighs.

5. Close your eyes and deepen your breath.

6. Breathe deeply in and out through your nose for 15 to 20 complete breaths.

7. To come out of the pose, slowly and gently open your eyes and release your hands down by your sides.

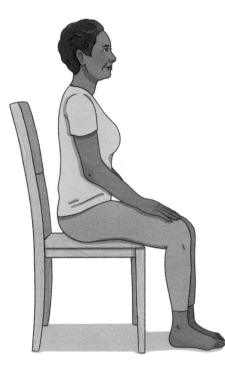

Tips

To add another element, try observing the way your abdomen moves in and out as you are breathing, or the way your chest expands with each inhale and contracts with each exhale.

Cautions

In case of lower-back or sits-bone pain from sitting on the hard surface of the chair, you can place a folded blanket between you and the seat for more cushioning.

Raised Hands Pose (Chair Urdhva Hastasana)

Body Areas Utilized: Arms, neck, shoulders, upper back

Good For: Warming up the upper back and increasing mobility in the shoulders

Instructions

1. Keep your body in the position of mountain pose by sitting up straight in your chair with your feet flat on the ground at hip-distance apart.

2. Take a deep inhale through your nose and bring your arms out and up above your head.

3. Keep your arms parallel to each other at shoulder-distance apart with your palms facing each other.

4. Look up toward your hands, keeping as much length as possible in the back of your neck.

5. On your next exhale, bring your hands outward and down by your sides with your palms facing your body. Bring your gaze back down to looking forward.

6. Repeat steps 2 through 5 four to eight times.

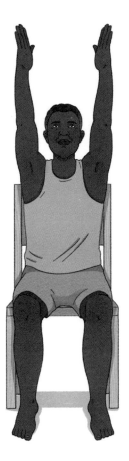

Tips

- Easier Variation: If you have trouble with shoulder mobility, you can keep your arms reaching out to the sides, parallel to the ground, instead of raising them all the way up.

- Challenging Variation: You can hold a yoga block in between your hands and raise the block from out in front of your body to reaching above your head.

Cautions

You may want to skip this pose if you are recovering from a shoulder, neck, or upper-back injury, or you have limited shoulder mobility.

Neck Rolls (Kantasanchalana)

Body Areas Utilized: Neck muscles

Good For: Gaining neck-joint mobility and muscle flexibility

Instructions

1. Remain sitting up tall in the chair with your palms on your thighs and your feet flat on the floor at hip-distance apart.

2. Inhale through your nose, then exhale through your nose while dropping your chin toward your chest.

3. Continue with your natural breath pattern, and gently rotate your head around, bringing your right ear toward your right shoulder. You don't need to rotate in time with your breath.

4. Continue the rotation, bringing your head around to the back, looking up toward the ceiling and keeping as much length in the back of your neck as possible.

5. Gently rotate your head around, bringing your left ear toward your left shoulder.

6. Bring your head back to the starting position with your chin toward your chest.

7. Repeat steps 3 through 6 eight to 10 times.

8. Repeat your rotations in the opposite direction eight to 10 times.

9. After your final rotation, gently bring your head back up, looking forward.

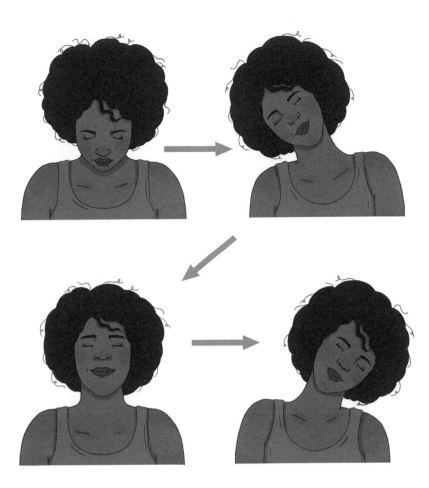

Tips

Easier Variation: You can forgo the rotations and simply tilt your head from side to side.

Cautions

You may want to skip this pose if you are recovering from a neck injury or if you have limited neck mobility.

Shoulder Rolls

Body Areas Utilized: Neck, shoulders, upper back

Good For: Releasing muscle tightness that comes from stress and tension and increasing mobility in the joints of the shoulders

Instructions

1. Remain sitting up tall in the chair with your palms on your thighs and your feet flat on the floor at hip-distance apart.

2. Inhale through your nose and raise both shoulders up toward your ears.

3. As you exhale, slowly and gently bring both shoulders toward the back of your body and then gently down and forward in a circular motion.

4. Continue the shoulder rotations in this direction in a smooth and gentle, continuous motion for eight to 10 rotations.

5. Repeat steps 2 and 3 in the opposite direction for eight to 10 rotations.

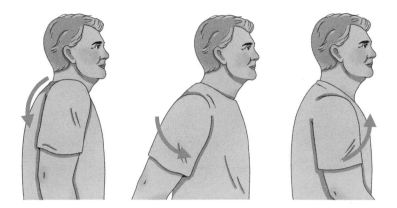

Tips

Easier Variation: You can raise your shoulders up toward your ears and back down in a shrugging motion instead of completing the rotations.

Cautions

You may want to skip this pose if you are recovering from a shoulder injury or if you have limited shoulder mobility. If you find difficulty when trying this pose, start with smaller shoulder circles and work toward making fuller circles.

Foot and Ankle Stretch

Body Areas Utilized: Ankles, feet, legs

Good For: Gaining joint mobility and muscle flexibility in the feet and ankles to help prevent pain while walking for long periods

Instructions

1. Sit up tall in the chair so that your back isn't leaning on the chair but is supported by your own strength, placing your feet flat on the floor at hip-distance apart.

2. Straighten your right leg out in front of you, placing your heel on the ground and flexing your foot.

3. Point your toes toward the floor, feeling a gentle stretch in the top of your foot.

4. Repeat flexing and pointing your foot 10 to 15 times and then gently bring your right leg back next to your left with your foot flat on the ground.

5. Repeat steps 2 through 4 with your left leg.

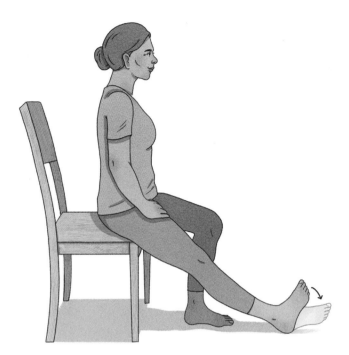

Tips

- Easier Variation: Keep your feet flat on the ground at hip-distance apart and raise your heel up and down, keeping your toes on the ground. Repeat on both sides.

- Challenging Variation: Instead of placing your foot on the ground, lift your foot two to three inches off the ground, keeping it elevated as you flex and point your toes.

Cautions

Move slowly and gently with intention to avoid pain during this movement. You may want to skip this exercise if you are recovering from a leg, foot, or ankle injury, or if you have limited mobility in those areas.

Side Bending Pose

Body Areas Utilized: Arms, neck, shoulders, sides of torso

Good For: Gaining joint mobility and muscle flexibility in your upper body, shoulders, and arms

Instructions

1. Sit up tall in the chair with your palms on your thighs and your feet flat on the floor at hip-distance apart.

2. Keeping both sits bones on the seat of the chair, place your left hand on your right thigh, palm down, and reach your right hand up and over to the left while looking upward and slightly tilting your torso over to the left. You should feel a stretch on the right side of your torso.

3. Hold here for one deep and complete breath, and then slowly come back to a neutral position with your spine straight and arms down by your sides.

4. Repeat on the opposite side by placing the right hand on the left thigh, reaching the left arm up and over to the right, and slightly tilting your torso right.

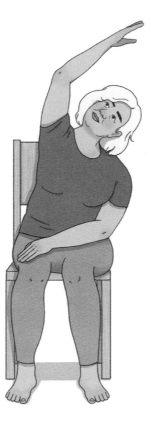

Tips

- Easier Variation: You can forgo the torso tilt and alternate raising your arms upward or out to the sides, depending on your flexibility.

- Challenging Variation: Instead of placing one hand on your thigh, you can try placing it behind you on the back of the chair, anywhere you can comfortably reach, for an additional shoulder and chest opening stretch.

Cautions

Try not to stretch too forcefully to avoid straining the muscles and causing pain in the side body. You may need to skip this pose if you're recovering from a back, arm, neck, or shoulder injury, or if you have limited mobility in those areas.

10-Minute Sequence at a Glance

On these two pages, you will see images of all the poses described in your 10-minute Warm-Up routine at a glance so you can easily reference them while you practice.

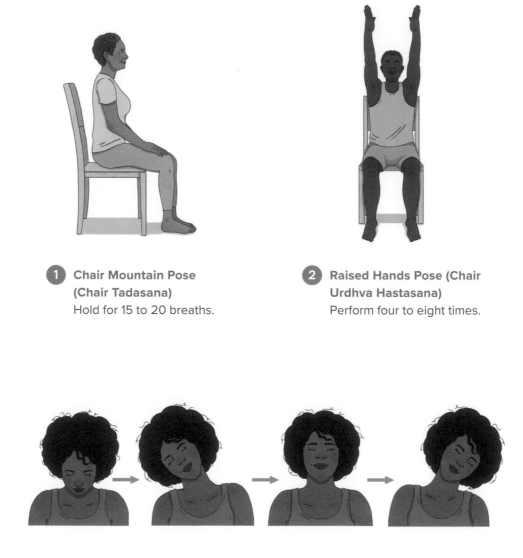

1 **Chair Mountain Pose (Chair Tadasana)**
Hold for 15 to 20 breaths.

2 **Raised Hands Pose (Chair Urdhva Hastasana)**
Perform four to eight times.

3 **Neck Rolls (Kantasanchalana)**
Repeat eight to 10 times for both directions.

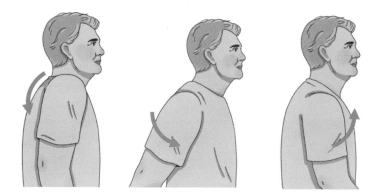

4 **Shoulder Rolls**
Repeat eight to 10 times for both directions.

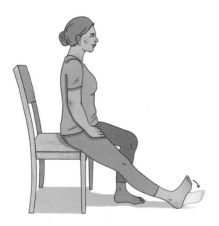

5 **Foot and Ankle Stretch**
Repeat 10 to 15 times on
each side.

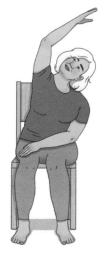

6 **Side Bending Pose**
Hold for one deep breath on
each side.

Reaching Energy

In yoga practice, you'll find that you are often instructed to "reach energy" through a particular body part or in a certain direction. This simply means exerting or focusing effort and maintaining continued alertness and attentiveness within the instructed body part or direction. It means that you shouldn't remain passive in this pose, but always have an element of activeness by continually reaching. This doesn't mean that you should be too forceful with your reaching—just a gentle and subtle focus of your internal energy will do.

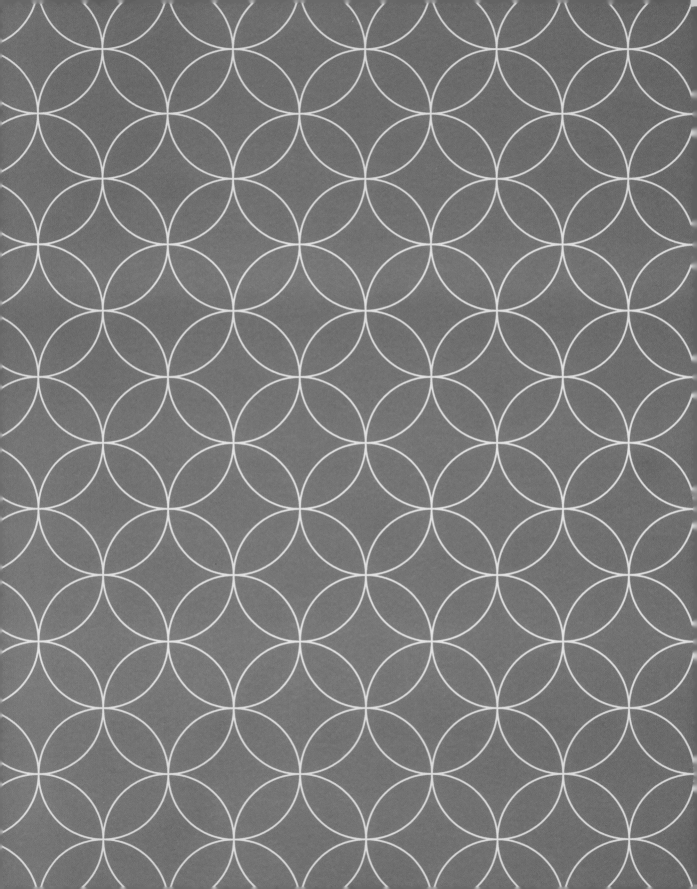

BEGIN GENTLY

In this chapter, you'll find chair yoga poses created for the yoga beginner or for people who need to be gentle with their movements due to injury, mobility issues, age, or illness. If you're looking to slowly improve mobility and flexibility or gain a bit more balance, these sequences are a great place for you to start. You can also turn to these routines as a way to gradually build strength in your body.

These poses are simple and easy to follow. They are a perfect way to begin your chair yoga journey while being very kind and gentle with yourself. Try out the following sequences as stand-alone routines or in combination with the 10-minute warm-up sequence from the previous chapter.

Chair Warrior 1 (Virabhadrasana 1)

Body Areas Utilized: Arms, neck, shoulders, upper back

Good For: Gaining flexibility and mobility in the shoulders, arms, and upper back, which will help alleviate tension in those areas so you can move more freely in your daily activities

Instructions

1. Sit up tall in the chair with your palms on your thighs and your feet flat on the floor at hip-distance apart.

2. Take a deep inhale through your nose and bring your arms out and up above your head.

3. Place your palms to meet each other above your head.

4. Look up toward your hands, keeping as much length as possible in the back of your neck.

5. Hold there for three to five deep inhales and exhales while reaching energy upward through your fingertips.

6. On your next exhale, bring your hands outward and down by your sides with your palms facing your body. Bring your gaze back down to looking forward.

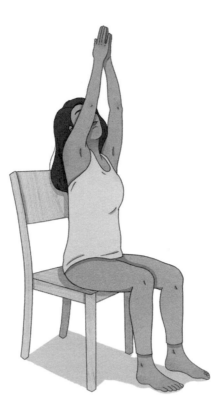

Tips

- Easier Variation: If you are struggling with mobility, you do not have to place your hands together above your head. You can keep your palms facing each other in front of you, shoulder-distance apart.

- Challenging Variation: For an upper-back stretch and chest opener, you can add a slight arch to your back by reaching your fingertips slightly up and backward on the diagonal.

Cautions

Be mindful not to scrunch your shoulders when looking upward, and instead relax them down away from your neck. If you are recovering from an injury in the back, shoulders, neck, or arms, then you may need to avoid this pose.

Seated Forward Bend (Paschimottanasana)

Body Areas Utilized: Back, hips, legs

Good For: Gaining flexibility and mobility in the hips and lower back, which often carry a lot of tension from stress and anxiety within our daily lives

Instructions

1. Sit up tall in the chair with your palms on your thighs and your feet flat on the floor at hip-distance apart.

2. Inhale through your nose while lengthening your spine and, on your exhale, drop your torso down so your belly is resting on your thighs.

3. Bring your hands down to the floor.

4. Relax your neck, allowing your head to release and hang down.

5. Hold here for three to five deep breaths.

6. To come up, gently press your hands into the ground and slowly lift your torso back up to a seated position.

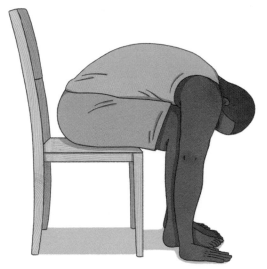

Tips

- Easier Variation: You can tilt forward halfway and place your hands on your knees for support instead of bending all the way to place your belly on your thighs.

- Challenging Variation: Bend your arms and hold on to opposite elbows, allowing your entire upper body to hang freely over your legs instead of planting your hands on the ground.

Cautions

You can always place your hands on an elevated surface, such as yoga blocks, to help alleviate some pain you may experience during this pose. If you are recovering from an injury or have limited mobility in the back, hips, or neck, you may need to avoid this pose.

Easy Seated Twist (Parivrtta Sukhasana)

Body Areas Utilized: Back, neck, arms

Good For: Gaining mobility in the spine and neck joints and increasing flexibility in the surrounding muscles, which can become tight due to stress, trauma, or injury

Instructions

1. Sit up tall in the chair with your palms on your thighs and your feet flat on the floor at hip-distance apart.

2. Bring your left hand to your right thigh and your right arm behind you on the seat of the chair.

3. Inhale and lengthen the spine, and on your exhale, gently twist your upper body around to the right, looking as far behind you as possible without straining yourself.

4. Remain here for eight to 10 deep breaths.

5. Gently unwind from your twist by coming back to center and bringing your arms down by your sides.

6. Repeat steps 2 through 5 on the opposite side.

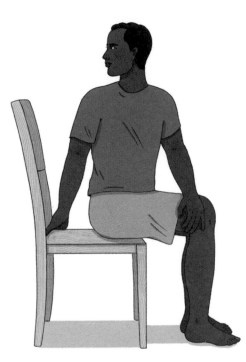

Tips

- Easier Variation: You can keep your gaze looking over to the side instead of trying to look all the way behind you. This will provide you with less of a twist in the spine.

- Challenging Variation: Try deepening your twist slightly with each exhale while you are holding the pose.

Cautions

Twisting can be challenging if you are pregnant, recovering from an injury, or have limited mobility in your back and neck, so you may want to work with caution or skip this pose. If you choose to try it, please twist very gently and be kind to your body.

Assisted Neck Stretch

Body Areas Utilized: Neck, shoulders

Good For: Gaining flexibility and mobility in the neck muscles and joints, and releasing stress and tension

Instructions

1. Sit up tall in the chair with your feet flat on the floor at hip-distance apart.

2. Gently tilt your head over to the right, keeping your shoulders even with each other.

3. Lightly wrap your right hand over the top of your head, helping to tilt it over and stretch the left side of your neck. Be careful not to pull too forcefully.

4. Hold for eight to 10 deep breaths.

5. Slowly release your hand and bring your head back upright.

6. Repeat steps 2 through 5 on the other side.

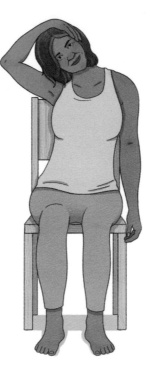

- Easier Variation: Just tilt your head without applying pressure with your hand.

Cautions

Please do not do this pose if you are recovering from a neck or shoulder injury, or if you have pain when moving and stretching the neck. The neck is very sensitive, and you want to allow it to completely heal before you stretch it in this way.

10-Minute Sequence at a Glance

On these two pages, you will see images of all the poses described in your 10-minute Begin Gently sequence at a glance so you can easily reference them while you practice.

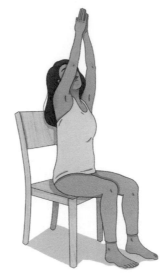

1 **Chair Warrior 1 (Virabhadrasana 1)**
Hold for three to five breaths. Perform two to four times.

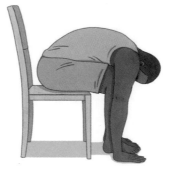

2 **Seated Forward Bend (Paschimottanasana)**
Hold for three to five breaths. Perform two to four times.

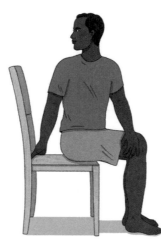

 Easy Seated Twist (Parivrtta Sukhasana)
Hold for eight to 10 breaths on each side.

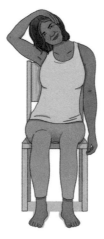

 Assisted Neck Stretch
Hold for eight to 10 breaths on each side.

Chair Cat/Cow (Chair Marjaryasana Bitilasana)

Body Areas Utilized: Back, neck, shoulders

Good For: Warming up the body and gaining mobility in the spine and flexibility in the muscles of the back

Instructions

1. Sit up tall in the chair with your palms on your thighs and your feet flat on the floor at hip-distance apart.

2. Bring your hands to your knees and on your inhale, using your hands to help move your chest forward, bring your back into a slight arch while looking upward.

3. On your next exhale, use your hands on your knees to help you curve your spine in the opposite direction, reaching your upper back toward the back of the chair and looking down toward the seat of the chair.

4. Repeat steps 2 through 3 for eight to 10 repetitions.

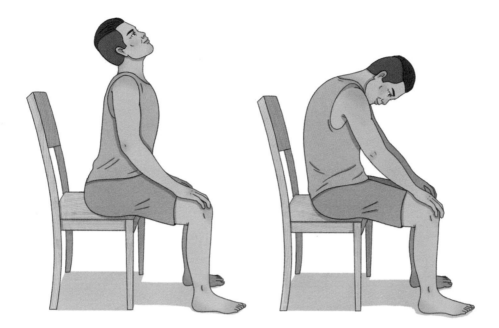

Tips

Challenging Variation: During cat pose (when your back is arched), pull gently on the backs of your thighs to increase the stretch.

Cautions

You may want to avoid this pose if you are recovering from a back injury or have limited mobility in that area. If you do try it, please move slowly, gently, and with intention. Don't be too forceful with your movements.

Cross-Legged Side Bend

....

Body Areas Utilized: Arms, obliques, thighs

Good For: Stretching and lengthening the sides of your torso, and feeling a gentle stretch in the sides of your thighs

....

Instructions

1. Sit up tall in the chair with your palms on your thighs and your feet flat on the floor at hip-distance apart.

2. Cross your right leg on top of your left leg.

3. Bring your left hand to your right thigh and reach your right arm up and over to the left, stretching the right side of your upper body.

4. Keep both sits bones even on the chair.

5. Hold for eight to 10 deep breaths.

6. Repeat steps 2 through 5 on the other side.

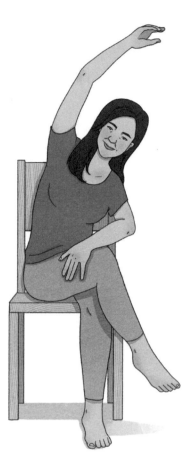

Tips

- Easier Variation: Complete the side stretch without crossing your legs.

- Challenging Variation: Instead of placing your hand on your leg, place it on the chair behind you for an additional chest opening and shoulder stretch.

Cautions

You may want to skip this pose if you are recovering from a back or shoulder injury, or if you have limited mobility in those areas.

Extended Chair Mountain Pose (Utthita Tadasana)

Body Areas Utilized: Neck, upper back, shoulders

Good For: Gaining flexibility and mobility in the chest, upper back, shoulders, and neck

Instructions

1. Sit up tall in the chair with your palms on your thighs and your feet flat on the floor at hip-distance apart.

2. Place the tips of your fingers on the seat of the chair behind you with the tops of your hands facing the back of the chair.

3. Take a deep inhale through your nose and look upward, reaching the center of your chest up and opening your shoulders apart from each other simultaneously.

4. Press down into your fingertips and rebound up through the center of your chest, reaching upward.

5. Remain here for three to five deep breaths.

6. Slowly come back to sitting upright and bring your hands down by your sides.

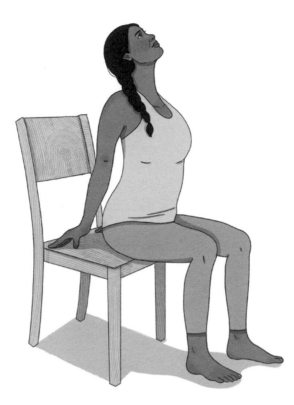

Tips

- Easier Variation: Keep your hands flat on your thighs and look up, coming into a very slight arch.

- Challenging Variation: Hold on to the sides of the back of the chair for a deeper arch and back stretch.

Cautions

This pose can be challenging for those who are recovering from a back, neck, or shoulder injury, or have limited mobility in those areas, so you may want to work with caution or skip this pose completely.

Single Leg Stretch (Janu Sirsasana)

. . . .

Body Areas Utilized: Hamstrings, hips, lower back

Good For: Gaining muscle flexibility and joint mobility in the hamstrings and hips—it feels great to release tension from these areas

. . . .

Instructions

1. Sit up tall in the chair with your palms on your thighs and your feet flat on the floor at hip-distance apart.

2. Straighten your right leg out in front of you, placing your heel on the ground and keeping your foot flexed.

3. Inhale and lengthen your spine, then exhale while bending your torso over and place both hands gently on the thigh or shin of your straightened leg.

4. Look down toward your leg and keep as much length in your spine as possible while bending forward.

5. Hold for three to five deep breaths.

6. Gently press into your hands to lift your spine back upright to a seated position and bring your hands down by your sides.

7. Repeat steps 2 through 6 on the opposite side.

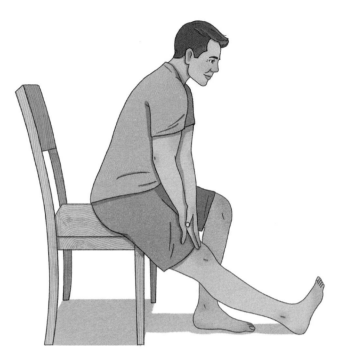

Tips

- Easier Variation: Keep your head looking forward instead of down toward your leg for less of a deep bend.

- Challenging Variation: If you are able to, hold on to your foot in your forward bend or you can place a strap around the foot and hold on to the strap for a deeper bend.

Cautions

You may want to skip this pose if you are recovering from an injury or have decreased mobility in the hamstrings, back, shoulders, or neck. Reaching forward with your leg stretched out can add an element of strain to those body parts because it can be a deeper stretch, so please be careful.

Chair Pigeon Pose (Eka Pada Rajakapotasana)

Body Areas Utilized: Hamstrings, hips, lower back, thighs

Good For: Gaining flexibility and mobility in the hips, hamstrings, and lower back, and alleviating pain from sciatica or any irritation of the sciatic nerve

Instructions

1. Sit up tall in the chair with your palms on your thighs and your feet flat on the floor at hip-distance apart.

2. Bending the right leg, cross your right ankle over your left thigh, keeping your right knee out to the side.

3. Place your right hand on your right shin just past your knee and your left hand on your right ankle, then gently tilt your torso forward while keeping your spine straight.

4. Hold for three to five deep breaths.

5. Press into your hands and gently bring your torso back to sitting upright.

6. Uncross your right leg and set it back down onto the ground.

7. Repeat steps 2 through 6 on the opposite side.

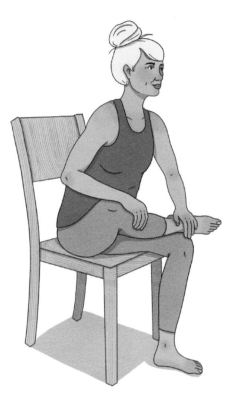

Tips

- Easier Variation: Cross your entire leg over your thigh and tilt your torso forward for a less intense leg and hip stretch.

- Challenging Variation: Bring your hands down to the ground or on top of yoga blocks for a deeper forward bend.

Cautions

You may want to skip this pose if you are recovering from an injury in the back, hamstrings, or hips, or if you have limited mobility in those areas or experience any degree of pain from this pose in your knee or hip joint.

Cross-Legged Twist (Parivrtta Sukhasana)

Body Areas Utilized: Back, hips, legs

Good For: Gaining muscle flexibility and joint mobility in the spine and hips—the twisting motion of this pose will help relieve tension and stiffness

Instructions

1. Sit up tall in the chair with your palms on your thighs and your feet flat on the floor at hip-distance apart.

2. Cross your entire right leg on top of your left thigh.

3. Place your left hand on your right thigh and place your right hand on the chair seat behind you.

4. Inhale and lengthen your spine, then exhale and twist your upper body around to the right, looking as far behind you as you can.

5. Hold for three to five deep breaths.

6. Slowly unwind from your twist, coming back to the center and uncrossing your leg, then placing it back down onto the ground.

7. Repeat steps 2 through 6 on the opposite side.

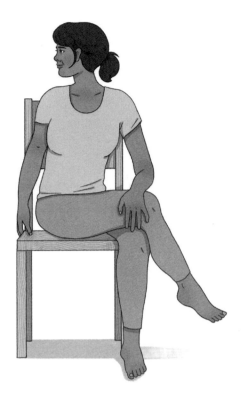

Tips

- Easier Variation: Keep your legs uncrossed and twist your upper body instead to lessen the intensity of the stretch.

- Challenging Variation: On each exhale, deepen your twist slightly by looking farther behind you.

Cautions

You may want to skip this step if you are recovering from an injury or have limited mobility in the back, neck, hips, legs, shoulders, or neck. Avoid twisting poses when you are pregnant or in the initial recovery stages of injury in these particular areas. Please allow your body to heal completely so you don't experience any pain while performing this pose.

Seated Forward Bend with Reach-Through Variation (Paschimottanasana)

Body Areas Utilized: Back, hips, legs

Good For: Gaining flexibility and mobility in the hips and lower back

Instructions

1. Sit up tall in the chair with your palms on your thighs and your feet flat on the floor a little wider than hip-distance apart.

2. Inhale and lengthen your spine, then exhale, dropping your torso down so your belly is resting on your upper thighs.

3. Bring your hands down to the floor and reach them in between your feet toward the rear legs of the chair, with the palms of your hands on the ground.

4. Relax your head and allow it to release and hang down.

5. Hold here for three to five deep breaths.

6. To come up, gently bring your hands forward and allow yourself to return to an upright position.

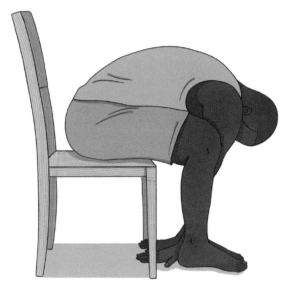

Tips

- Easier Variation: Keep your hands directly underneath your shoulders or place them on yoga blocks instead of reaching them back.

- Challenging Variation: Place your palms flat on the ground with your elbows bent at a 90-degree angle and pointed toward the rear chair legs.

Cautions

You may want to skip this pose if you are recovering from an injury or have limited mobility in the back, hips, or neck. If you do try it, don't force yourself; you can still benefit from the pose even if your bend is slight.

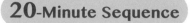

Chair Corpse Pose (Chair Savasana)

Body Areas Utilized: Back

Good For: Relaxing, calming down, and unwinding at the end of your practice

Instructions

1. Sit up tall in the chair with your back resting on the back of the chair, your palms facing upward on your thighs, and your feet flat on the floor at hip-distance apart.

2. Close your eyes, focus your attention inward, and deepen your breathing.

3. Breathing in and out through your nose, begin to draw your attention to your breath.

4. Focus on your inhales and exhales.

5. You can count your breaths, notice your breath, or feel your chest and abdomen moving in and out as you breathe.

6. Remain here for 25 to 30 deep rounds of breathing.

7. When you are ready, slowly and gently open your eyes.

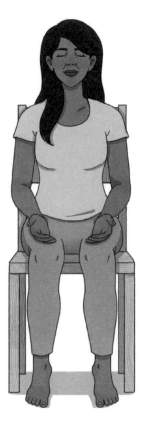

Tips

- Easier Variation: Lie flat on the ground without a chair if that is more comfortable, or place a folded blanket on the seat of the chair.

- Challenging Variation: If you are able to, lie flat on the ground facing the chair and place your calves on top of the seat of the chair. Lay your hands on the ground down by your sides with your palms facing upward.

Cautions

If sitting for long periods of time is uncomfortable for you, lessen the time you remain in this pose. You'll benefit more by doing it for a short duration than risking aggravating your sensitive joints or muscles by staying in the pose too long.

20-Minute Sequence at a Glance

On these two pages, you will see images of all the poses described in your 20-minute Begin Gently sequence at a glance so you can easily reference them while you practice.

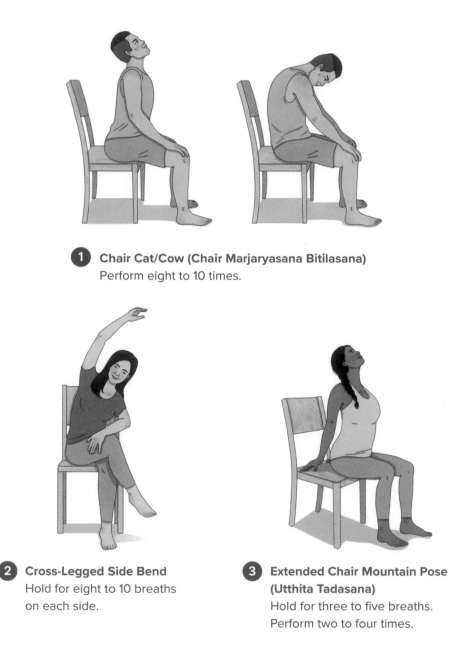

1 **Chair Cat/Cow (Chair Marjaryasana Bitilasana)**
Perform eight to 10 times.

2 **Cross-Legged Side Bend**
Hold for eight to 10 breaths on each side.

3 **Extended Chair Mountain Pose (Utthita Tadasana)**
Hold for three to five breaths. Perform two to four times.

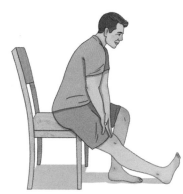

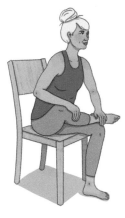

4 **Single Leg Stretch (Janu Sirsasana)**
Hold for three to five breaths on each side.

5 **Chair Pigeon Pose (Eka Pada Rajakapotasana)**
Hold for three to five breaths on each side.

6 **Cross-Legged Twist (Parivrtta Sukhasana)**
Hold for three to five breaths on each side.

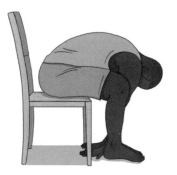

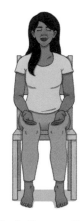

7 **Seated Forward Bend with Reach-Through Variation (Paschimottanasana)**
Hold for three to five breaths. Perform two to four times.

8 **Chair Corpse Pose (Chair Savasana)**
Hold for 25 to 30 breaths.

Yoga for the Face

Face yoga isn't traditional to a yoga practice, but it has been gaining popularity as a way to increase circulation, strengthen facial muscles, and bring more blood flow to the eyes and brain. Some people have also found it helpful in combatting TMJ (temporomandibular joint) dysfunction, migraines, and eye strain. Face yoga is something that you can try anytime and it's fairly simple.

One simple exercise you can try involves your mouth. You can keep your eyes open or closed, whichever you feel more comfortable doing. Take a deep inhale through your nose, and on the exhale, blow out a "raspberry" through your mouth. If you can, try to involve your cheeks in the exhale as well and notice the vibration of your lips as the exhale is being released. You can repeat this from one to three times per day to release and stress or tension.

Another exercise you can try is a stretch for your neck and throat area. Tip your head backward until you feel a stretch in the front of your neck and throat area. Alternate between opening your mouth, pursing your lips, and sticking your tongue out, holding each one for about five seconds each. You can repeat this up to three times.

Incorporating face yoga into your daily routine can be a fun and interesting way to relieve some tension and improve your health in that area of the body.

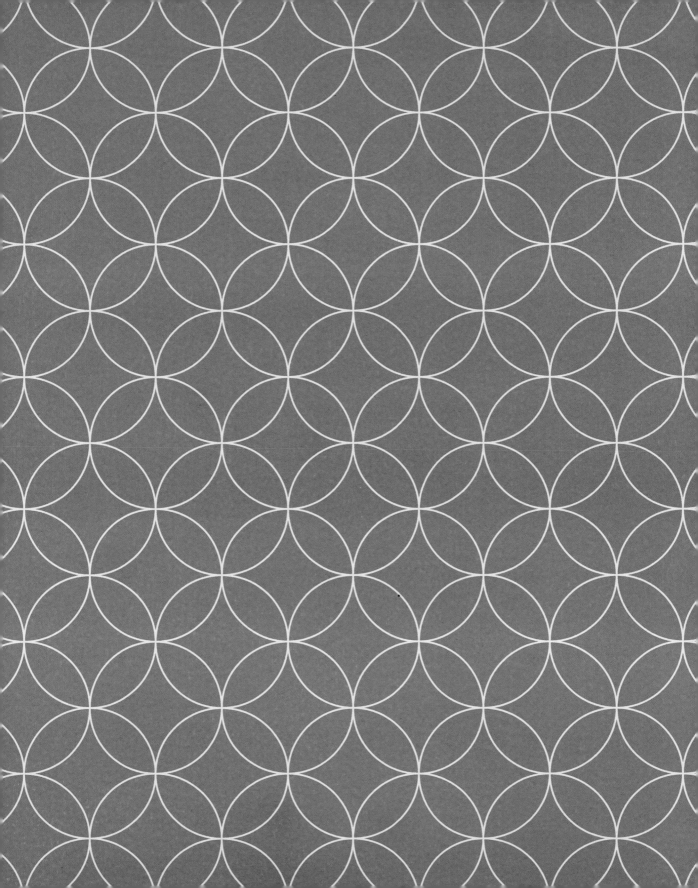

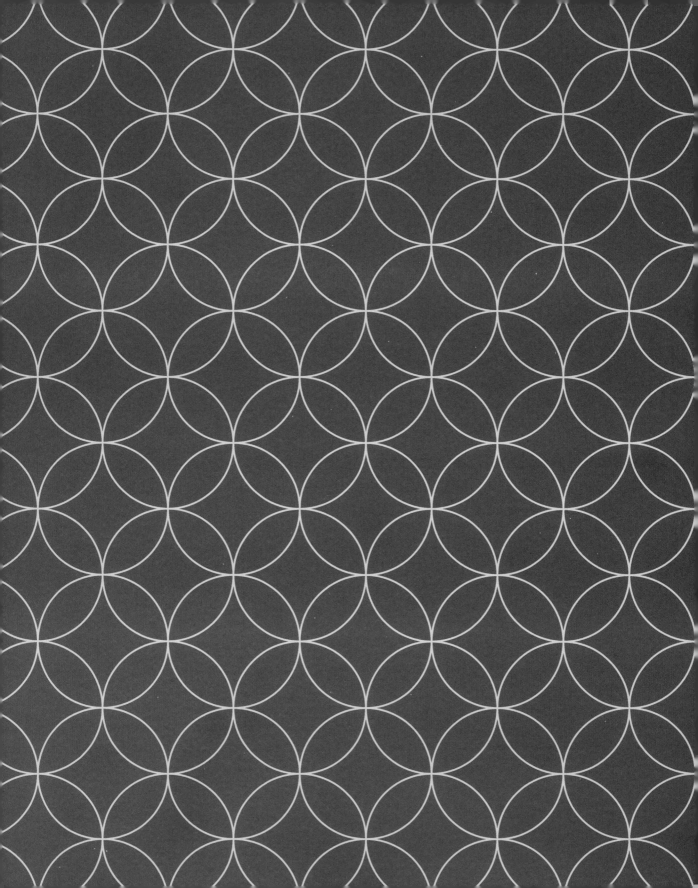

TONE AND FLOW

In this chapter, I am sharing two chair yoga routines that are slightly more dynamic and tailored to the intermediate level. Once you're ready, you can use these sequences to enhance your chair yoga practice and add some more challenging elements. These routines can be used after the warm-up routines (or a series of warm-up poses) once your body is ready to go.

Because the poses in these sequences are more challenging, some of them do involve standing beside the chair. But if you are unable to stand, perhaps you can try the poses in this sequence where you remain seated. Whether you're sitting down or standing up, these poses will add more variety into your practice and you'll be able to work on your strength, flexibility, and stamina. You might even break a sweat!

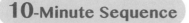

Knee to Chest Pose (Eka Pada Apanasana)

Body Areas Utilized: Abdominals, hips, hamstrings

Good For: Gaining hip and hamstring flexibility and gently strengthening the abdominals

Instructions

1. Sit up tall in the chair with your feet flat on the ground at hip-distance apart.

2. Lift your right leg, bend your knee, and hold on to your shin with both hands.

3. Flex your right foot.

4. Hold here for three to five deep inhales and exhales.

5. Gently release your foot back down to the ground.

6. Repeat steps 2 through 5 with your left leg.

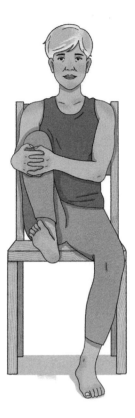

Tips

- Easier Variation: Hold on to the hamstrings instead of the shin, and you can also place a support such as stacked yoga blocks under your lifted leg, if needed.

- Challenging Variation: Flow between flexing and pointing the foot while holding this pose on each side.

Cautions

You may want to skip this pose if you are recovering from a hamstring, hip, or knee injury, because it could cause more pain in that area.

Opposite Leg and Knee Lift (Vyaghrasana Variation)

Body Areas Utilized: Abdominals, hamstrings, hips, quadriceps

Good For: Strengthening the hips, quadriceps, and abdominals—it's also helpful for stretching the hip joint, making it easier to walk and bend down. Stretching this muscle group also helps to alleviate tension in that area, making it more comfortable when seated

Instructions

1. Begin with both feet flat on the ground at hip-distance apart, sitting up tall in the chair.

2. Lift your right foot four to six inches off of the ground, keeping your foot flexed and parallel to the floor.

3. Reach your left arm out in front of you with your palm facing upward.

4. Engage your abdominal muscles and hold this pose for three to five deep inhales and exhales.

5. Gently release your arm and leg back down.

6. Repeat steps 2 through 5 on the opposite side.

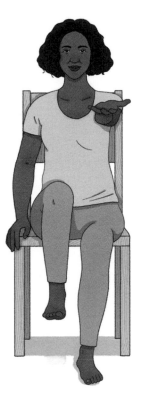

Tips

- Easier Variation: Hold on to the side of the chair as you lift your leg up and hold there, or use a support such as stacked yoga blocks under your raised leg, if needed.

- Challenging Variation: Try straightening your raised leg out in front of you, keeping your leg parallel to the ground or lower.

Cautions

You may want to skip this pose if you are recovering from a hip, hamstring, or quadricep injury, because it may be challenging for you to lift your leg in that way.

Chair Boat Pose (Chair Navasana)

Body Areas Utilized: Abdominals, hamstrings, hips, quadriceps

Good For: Strengthening the abdominals, hips, and quadriceps, as you are required to hold your legs up using your abdominal muscles

Instructions

1. Sit up tall in the chair with your feet flat on the ground at hip-distance apart.

2. Lean your back against the back of the chair, engage your abdominal muscles, and lift your legs about 12 inches off the ground, one leg at a time, keeping your feet flexed.

3. Place your hands on the top of your thighs.

4. Hold here with your legs raised for three to five deep breaths.

5. Gently release each leg down to the ground, one at a time.

6. Repeat steps 2 through 5 twice more.

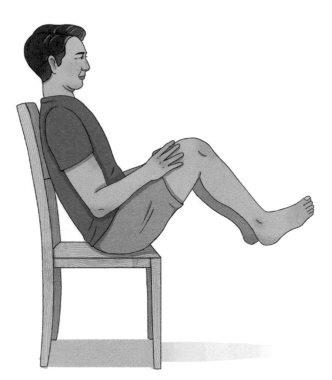

Tips

- Easier Variation: Place your feet on stacked yoga blocks and hold the pose there. Just make sure your torso is leaning slightly back at a tilt. You can hold on to the chair for support.

- Challenging Variation: Try straightening your legs, bringing your body into a V-shape. You can also try reaching your arms forward toward your feet and keeping them straight as you hold the pose.

Cautions

You will want to avoid doing this pose if you are recovering from an injury in your abdominals, hips, or quadriceps. This is a quite challenging pose, so if you choose to try it, please be careful.

Chair Forward Bending Twist (Chair Parivrtta Uttanasana)

Body Areas Utilized: Arms, back, hamstrings, hips

Good For: Stretching the hamstrings, hips, and spine and gaining flexibility in the muscles of those areas—you'll also gently strengthen the muscles in the raised arm

Instructions

1. Begin sitting in the chair with your feet flat on the floor at hip-distance apart.

2. Inhale and lengthen your spine, then exhale and fold your torso over your legs, bringing your left hand down to the ground by your feet and lifting your right arm to reach up toward the ceiling.

3. Your torso should be facing your right leg.

4. Hold here for three to five deep breaths.

5. Gently unwind from your twist and bring your torso back upright.

6. Repeat steps 2 through 5 on the opposite side.

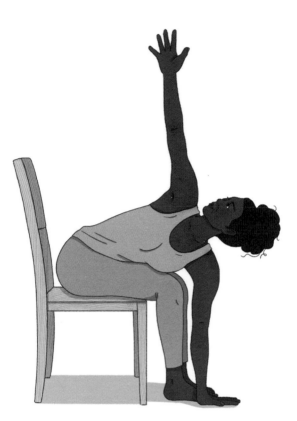

Tips

- Easier Variation: Place your bottom hand on your leg or on stacked yoga blocks to lessen the intensity of the forward fold.

- Challenging Variation: Try bending your raised arm and placing your hand behind your back for a deeper chest-opening stretch.

Cautions

If you are pregnant or recovering from a back, neck, hip, or hamstring injury, you will want to avoid this pose. Always work with caution when trying any twisting pose and twist very gently to avoid any muscle strain or joint pain.

Chair Tree Pose (Chair Vrksasana)

....

Body Areas Utilized: Arms, core, legs

Good For: Strengthening your legs and improving your balance, which can make it easier for you to go about your everyday life

....

Instructions

1. Stand up behind the chair with the left side of your body facing the back of the chair.

2. Hold on to the chair with your left hand and raise your right leg off the ground.

3. Place the bottom of your right foot against your inner left leg under the knee joint. Don't place your foot on your knee.

4. Raise your right arm above your head. You can also place your right hand on your right hip for variation.

5. Hold this pose for six to eight deep breaths.

6. Gently release your hand and foot down.

7. Repeat steps 1 through 6 on the opposite side.

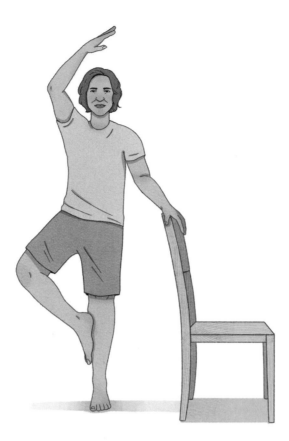

- Easier Variation: Substitute this pose with Raised Hands Pose (page 12) when you are practicing the full sequence.

- Challenging Variation: Place your raised foot on your inner thigh if your flexibility allows you to do so. You can also try lifting one or both of your arms to reach up toward the ceiling.

Cautions

If you are recovering from a leg, foot, ankle, or hip injury, or are experiencing pain in those areas, then you will likely want to avoid this pose. If you do try this pose, the raised foot may shift while you are trying to gain your balance at times, so always be cautious of not placing your foot on your knee joint.

Dangling Pose (Uttanasana Variation)

Body Areas Utilized: Back, hamstrings, hips

Good For: Stretching and finding length and space in the spine, as well as gaining muscle flexibility in the hips and hamstrings

Instructions

1. Stand up tall, facing your body away from the chair with your feet at hip-distance apart and parallel to each other.

2. Place your hands on your hips, bend your knees, and gently fold your torso over your legs from your hips with a straight spine.

3. Once your torso is as far down as your flexibility will allow, take hold of opposite elbows in both of your hands.

4. Allow your head, neck, and spine to gently hang down toward the ground and release.

5. Hold here for six to eight deep breaths.

6. To come up, place your hands on your hips, and return to standing with bent knees and a straight spine.

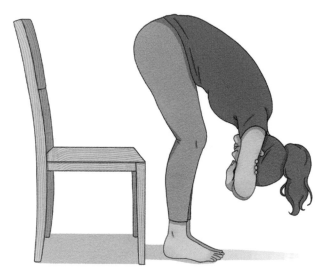

Tips

- Easier Variation: Keep your hands on the ground or on stacked yoga blocks if the stretch feels too intense. You can also keep your knees bent.

- Challenging Variation: Try wrapping your arms around your legs and gently pulling your upper body toward your thighs.

Cautions

You will want to skip this pose if you are recovering from a hip, hamstring, back, or neck injury, because it could cause some pain in those areas. The weight of your head as it is released downward can be too heavy for a recovering neck, so if you do try this pose, please be careful.

10-Minute Sequence at a Glance

On these two pages, you will see images of all the poses described in your 10-minute Tone and Flow sequence at a glance so you can easily reference them while you practice.

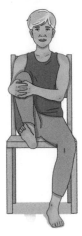

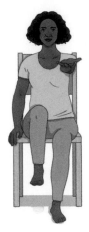

1 **Knee to Chest Pose (Eka Pada Apanasana)**
Hold for three to five breaths on each side.

2 **Opposite Leg and Knee Lift (Vyaghrasana Variation)**
Hold for three to five breaths on each side.

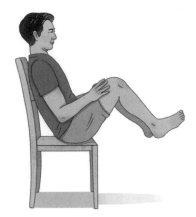

3 **Chair Boat Pose (Chair Navasana)**
Hold for three to five breaths. Perform three times.

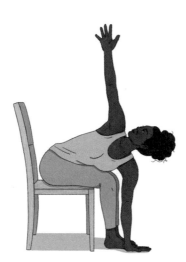

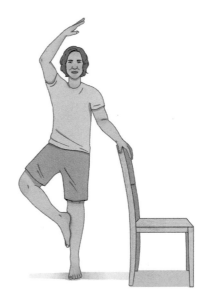

4 Chair Forward Bending Twist
(Chair Parivrtta Uttanasana)
Hold for three to five breaths on
each side.

5 Chair Tree Pose (Chair Vrksasana)
Hold for six to eight breaths on
each side.

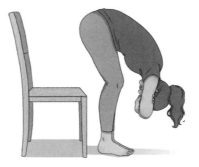

6 Dangling Pose (Uttanasana Variation)
Hold for six to eight breaths. Perform
two to four times.

Chair Goddess Pose (Chair Utkata Konasana)

Body Areas Utilized: Arms, hips, inner thighs

Good For: Gaining muscle flexibility in the inner thighs and strength in the arms

Instructions

1. Begin sitting up tall in the chair with your feet flat on the ground.

2. Bring your legs out wide so that one leg is on either side of the chair.

3. Reach your arms out to the side and bend both elbows, keeping your hands widely stretched and fingertips engaged.

4. Face your palms forward.

5. Hold here for six to eight deep breaths.

6. To release, bring your legs back to the center of the chair and your arms down by your sides.

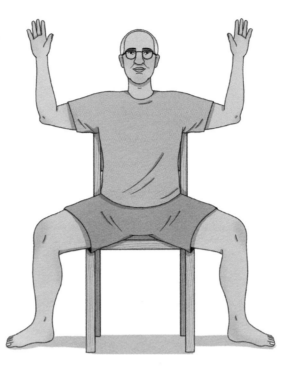

Tips

- Easier Variation: Keep your legs slightly closer together if the stretch in the inner thighs is too intense.

- Challenging Variation: Try raising your heels off the ground and holding the pose, or try the standing variation of this pose where you are not supporting your weight with the chair.

Cautions

You may want to skip this pose if you are recovering from an inner thigh, hip, or arm injury. The intensity of holding your body in this pose requires strength that an injury in those areas may have diminished. If you choose to give it a try, you can hold the pose for less time than instructed if it becomes too challenging for you.

Chair Goddess Twist (Chair Parivrtta Utkata Konasana)

Body Areas Utilized: Arms, hips, inner thighs, sides of torso

Good For: Stretching the oblique muscles and hips, strengthening the arm muscles, and boosting your mood and confidence

Instructions

1. Repeat the position of your legs from the previous Chair Goddess Pose (page 74).

2. Tilt your upper body over to the left, raising your right arm up toward the ceiling and your left arm down toward your left ankle.

3. Look up toward your right hand and keep your palms facing forward.

4. Hold this twist for three to five deep breaths.

5. Gently come back up to a seated position.

6. Repeat steps 2 through 5 on the opposite side.

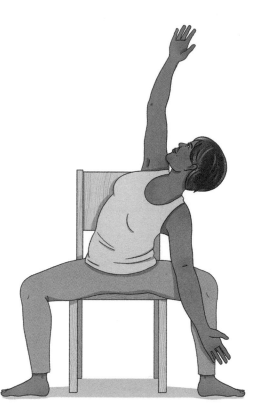

Tips

- Easier Variation: Place a support, such as a stack of yoga blocks, under the lower hand to lessen the intensity of the bend.

- Challenging Variation: Try bending the elbow of your raised arm and placing your hand behind your back for a deeper chest-opening stretch.

Cautions

If you are pregnant or recovering from a hip, back, or hamstring injury, you will likely want to avoid this pose. Twisting can be a bit challenging for the body regardless of whether or not you are recovering from an injury. If you choose to try it, you can lessen the intensity by not twisting as deeply or holding the pose for less time than instructed.

Chair Wide-Legged Forward Bend (Chair Prasarita Padottanasana)

Body Areas Utilized: Back, hamstrings, hips

Good For: Gaining muscle flexibility in the hamstrings, hips, and back, while also providing an element of relaxation due to the action of bending forward

Instructions

1. Bring your legs to the position of the previous two poses, Chair Goddess Pose (page 74) and Chair Goddess Twist (page 76).

2. Gently fold your torso down toward the ground, bringing your hands to the floor and allowing your head to hang down freely.

3. Hold here for six to eight deep breaths.

4. To come back up, gently and slowly bring your torso back upright with a straight spine.

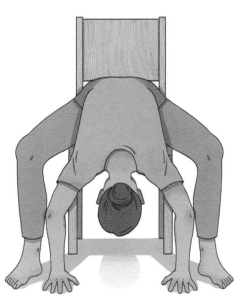

Tips

- Easier Variation: Place your hands on top of supports, such as stacked yoga blocks, to lessen the intensity of the bend.

- Challenging Variation: Try holding on to your ankles with both hands and gently pulling yourself into a deeper bend.

Cautions

You will likely want to skip this pose if you are recovering from a back, neck, hip, or hamstring injury. This pose can be relaxing, but the weight of your head can be too heavy for a recovering neck, so please be careful with your head and neck if you attempt this pose.

Eagle Arms
(Chair Garudasana)

Body Areas Utilized: Arms, upper back, shoulders

Good For: Stretching and gaining flexibility in the upper back, gaining shoulder mobility, and increasing focus and concentration

Instructions

1. Sit up tall in the chair with your feet flat on the floor parallel to each other at hip-distance apart.

2. Reach both your arms out to the side.

3. Bring them in front of your body, bend your elbows, and cross your upper arms so that your right arm is on top of your left arm.

4. Wrap your forearms around each other and bring your palms to meet in front of your face.

5. Keep your upper arms parallel to your thighs.

6. Hold here for six to eight deep breaths.

7. Release your arms from the cross and repeat steps 2 through 6 on the opposite side.

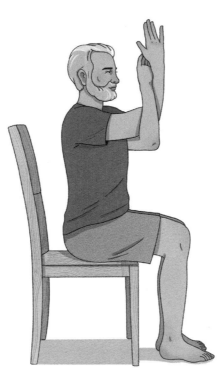

Tips

- Easier Variation: Instead of wrapping your upper arms around to make your palms meet, you can place the backs of your hands together.

- Challenging Variation: With your arms in this position, fold your torso forward, bringing your spine into a curve.

Cautions

You may want to skip this step if you are recovering from a back, arm, or shoulder injury, because it requires a bit of flexibility in those areas. If you are still recovering, you may need to work your way up to being able to practice this.

Chair Warrior 2 (Virabhadrasana 2)

Body Areas Utilized: Arms, hamstrings, hips, quadriceps

Good For: Strengthening the muscles in your arms and legs while also instilling a sense of confidence and power, as this is a very strong and engaging pose

Instructions

1. Begin sitting up tall in the chair.

2. Gently shift your body so that your right hamstring is flat on the chair's seat with your right knee bent over the side of the chair. Put your left leg straight out to the other side with your left foot flat on the floor at a 45-degree angle.

3. Reach both of your arms straight out to the side, keeping your palms facing down.

4. Look over your right hand and keep your gaze above it.

5. Hold here for three to five deep breaths.

6. Gently and slowly bring your body back to the center of the chair.

7. Repeat steps 2 through 6 on the opposite side.

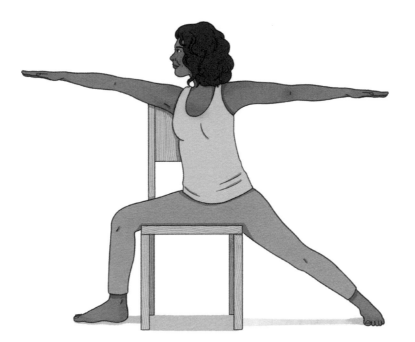

Tips

- Easier Variation: Just practice the arms and keep both sits bones on the chair with your legs parallel at hip-distance apart.

- Challenging Variation: Try the standing version of this pose where you are supporting your weight by standing. You can also hold on to the back of the chair while doing so for support.

Cautions

If you are recovering from a hip, back, or leg injury, you may want to avoid this pose. It requires a bit more energy and strength, which can be quite taxing on a recovering body. You can try holding the pose for less time than instructed, or you can try just the arm or just the leg portion depending on the specific location of your injury.

Chair Reverse Warrior (Chair Viparita Virabhadrasana)

Body Areas Utilized: Arms, back, hips, legs

Good For: Strengthening the muscles in your legs and stretching the muscles in the sides of your torso—the combination of strength and stretch can provide a calming energy to the body and mind

Instructions

1. Begin sitting up tall in the chair.

2. Gently shift your body so that your right hamstring is flat on the chair's seat with your right knee bent over the side of the chair. Put your left leg straight out to the other side with your left foot flat on the floor at a 45-degree angle.

3. Reach both of your arms straight out to the side, keeping your palms facing down.

4. Look over your right hand and keep your gaze above it.

5. Turn your right palm facing upward, and reach that arm forward, up, and back in an arcing motion.

6. Keep your right arm straight and reach it back toward the left leg on a diagonal.

7. Hold here for three to five deep breaths.

8. Gently bring your right arm back down and repeat steps 2 through 7 on the opposite side.

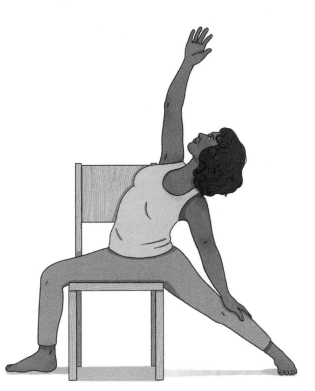

Tips

- Easier Variation: Complete the arm portion while keeping both of your legs on the chair's seat and hold on to the chair's side for support.

- Challenging Variation: Try the standing version of this pose with your weight fully supported by your legs. You can also hold on to the back of the chair for more support.

Cautions

If you are recovering from a hip, back, neck, leg, or arm injury, you will probably want to avoid this pose. It is one of the deeper back bends provided in this book, so be especially careful if your back is sensitive.

Chair Downward Dog (Adho Mukha Svanasana)

Body Areas Utilized: Arms, back, hips, legs

Good For: Improving your sense of balance and gaining back muscle flexibility and leg strength

Instructions

1. Stand up tall, facing the chair, with your feet parallel to each other at hip-distance apart.

2. Place both your hands on the chair's seat and make sure they feel stable.

3. Step your feet backward until you feel your spine is straightened.

4. Hold here for six to eight deep breaths.

5. Gently using the support of the chair on your hands, walk your feet back toward the chair and slowly come up to standing.

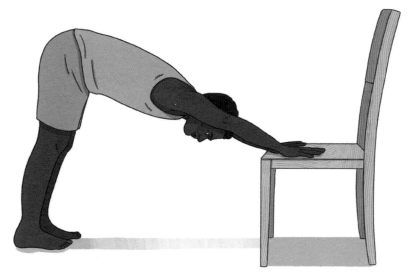

Tips

- Easier Variation: Try this pose with your hands on the back of the chair to lessen the intensity of the forward bend.

- Challenging Variation: Try bending your elbows and placing your forearms on the seat of the chair for a more intense arm-strengthening exercise.

Cautions

You will want to avoid this pose if you are recovering from a shoulder, arm, hand, wrist, leg, or hip injury. Most of your weight is being supported by your legs, so if you have trouble with standing due to a lower-body injury, definitely work with caution if attempting this pose.

Chair High Lunge

Body Areas Utilized: Arms, hamstrings, hips, legs, quadriceps

Good For: Strengthening the muscles in your legs and arms and gaining hip and hamstring muscle flexibility—it's a deep stretch that releases tension from those areas in a supportive way

Instructions

1. Stand to the side of the chair with the back of the chair to your left. Place your right foot on the chair.

2. Lean forward into your bent right leg so that your left leg is straight out behind you, keeping your left heel on the ground.

3. Place your left hand on the back of the chair for support and raise your right arm upward.

4. Hold here for three to five deep breaths.

5. To come out of the lunge, place your right foot back on the ground, bring your right arm down, and release your left hand from the chair.

6. Walk around to the other side of the chair and repeat steps 2 through 5 on the opposite side.

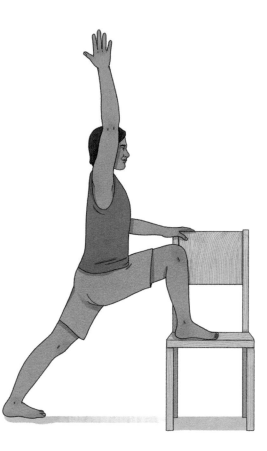

Tips

- Easier Variation: Stand behind the chair, facing the chair's back. Keep both legs straight and both feet on the ground at hip-distance apart, and place both your hands on the back of the chair for support as you bend forward, creating a flat back.

- Challenging Variation: Raise both arms up toward the ceiling instead of keeping one hand on the chair.

Cautions

If you are recovering from a leg, hip, arm, or shoulder injury, you will want to avoid this pose. The stretching of the hamstring and hips can be quite deep and intense in this pose, and if you choose to try it, don't lunge as far forward, which will help reduce the intensity.

Intense Side Stretch (Parsvottanasana)

Body Areas Utilized: Arms, back, hamstrings, hips, shoulders

Good For: Stretching the sides of your legs, gaining flexibility in the hips, and strengthening the legs—it's a deeper stretch that may be intense at first, but can help you move more freely in daily life

Instructions

1. Stand up tall facing the front of the chair's seat with your feet parallel to each other.

2. Step your right foot back and place it down about a leg's distance away from your left foot.

3. Bring your hands to your hips and slowly tilt your torso forward until it's parallel to the ground.

4. Place your hands on the seat of the chair, keeping your legs and spine straight and your neck in line with your spine.

5. Hold here for six to eight deep breaths.

6. Slowly bring your hands back to your hips and your torso back up to standing.

7. Bring your right foot forward to meet the left.

8. Repeat steps 2 through 7 on the opposite side.

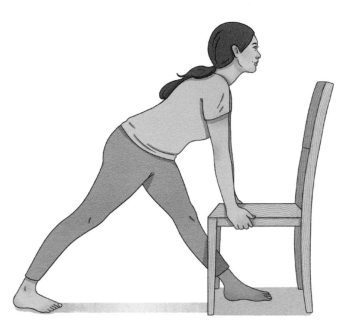

Tips

- Easier Variation: Keep your legs together in a parallel position and bring your hands to the seat of the chair for a forward bend.

- Challenging Variation: Instead of placing your hands on the seat of the chair, place them on the back of the chair for a slightly more intense shoulder stretch.

Cautions

You may want to avoid this pose if you are recovering from a back, neck, leg, hip, arm, or shoulder injury. This pose may look simple, but it can be quite challenging for the legs, so practice with caution if you are sensitive in the joints and muscles of the legs.

20-Minute Sequence at a Glance

On these two pages, you will see images of all the poses described in your 20-minute Tone and Flow sequence at a glance so you can easily reference them while you practice.

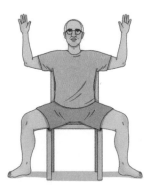

1 **Chair Goddess Pose (Chair Utkata Konasana)** Hold for six to eight breaths. Perform two to four times.

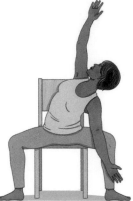

2 **Chair Goddess Twist (Chair Parivrtta Utkata Konasana)** Hold for three to five breaths on each side.

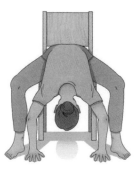

3 **Chair Wide-Legged Forward Bend (Chair Prasarita Padottanasana)** Hold for six to eight breaths. Perform two to four times.

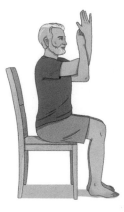

4 **Eagle Arms (Chair Garudasana)** Hold for six to eight breaths on each side.

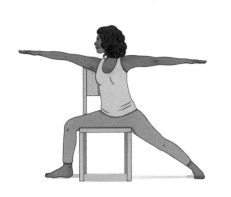

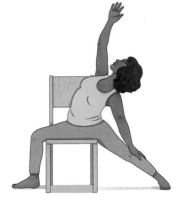

5 Chair Warrior 2 (Virabhadrasana 2)
Hold for three to five breaths on each side.

6 Chair Reverse Warrior (Chair Viparita Virabhadrasana)
Hold for three to five breaths on each side.

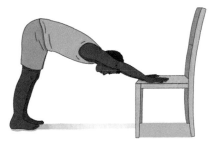

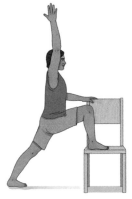

7 Chair Downward Dog (Adho Mukha Svanasana) Hold for six to eight breaths. Perform two to four times.

8 Chair High Lunge
Hold for three to five breaths on each side.

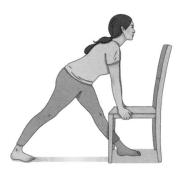

9 Intense Side Stretch (Parsvottanasana)
Hold for six to eight breaths on each side.

Yoga and Healing

Incorporating a regular yoga practice into your life is a great way to promote inner healing. As I discussed earlier, it not only helps with your physical body, but it can also greatly help your mental state. Even just incorporating only the physical yoga postures into your life without practicing meditation along with it can help you mentally as well, and your mental state affects your physical health and ability to heal.

According to ancient yogic belief systems, the mind is a powerful tool in healing and regenerating the body. When we are able to achieve the mental clarity and calmness that yoga provides, we often find that we have more awareness of our bodies, which can help us reduce pain. Mental clarity also provides you with a better ability to focus and concentrate on one task at a time. This enables you to better identify where your pain is coming from, which can ultimately help you focus on healing that area.

One thing that you can do while practicing yoga that can help you achieve mental clarity and calmness is to simply focus on each movement you are doing. Instead of coming into your yoga pose, settling there, and then focusing on what you are going to have for dinner, focus on your breath and how your body is feeling at that moment. If you are moving in the pose, focus on each and every movement you are doing. As your arms are lifting, notice the pathway that they are moving in and which muscles you are using to lift your arms. This is actually considered another form of meditation that you might find a little easier to start with than sitting still and focusing on your breath. Adding this element to your yoga practice will help you achieve more calmness and sharpen your sense of focus. Ultimately, you just may find that you start to feel better overall—not only mentally, but physically as well.

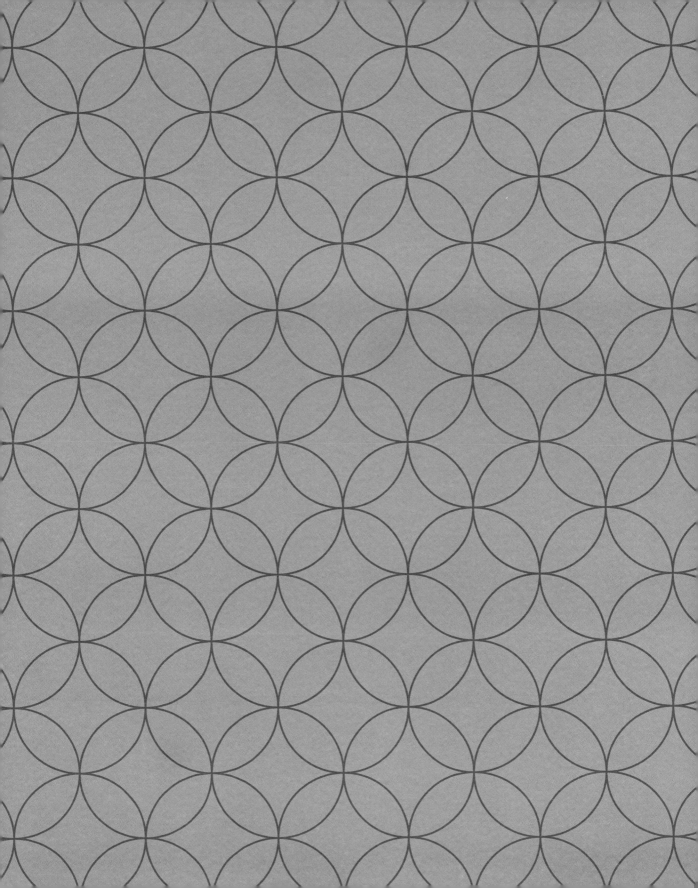

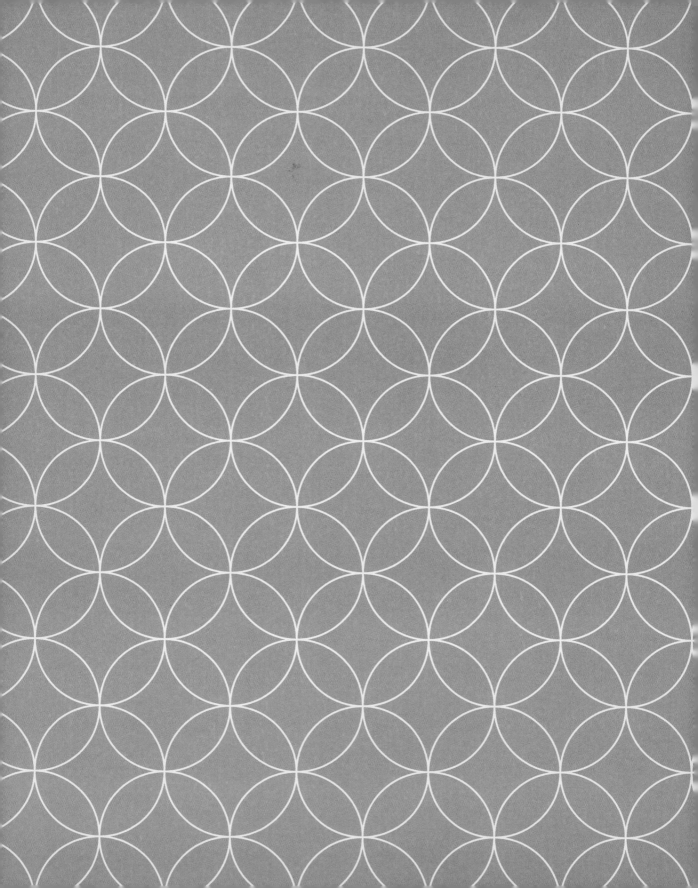

UNWIND AND SLEEP

In this chapter, I'll share two chair yoga routines that will help you relax, unwind, and sleep. These poses were inspired by the restorative yoga technique and have a more meditative and calming quality to them. You will be instructed to hold some of the poses for slightly longer than you have for the previous poses, which will allow you to enter the practice of mediation and focus your attention inward. Doing so will activate your parasympathetic nervous system, helping you feel calmer overall.

Some of these poses involve sitting or lying on the ground and using the chair as support for certain body parts. But if you are unable to do them, there are still plenty of poses in this chapter that involve being seated in the chair and will bring you the same benefits. There are definitely poses for everyone here, so try not to get discouraged by the look of certain poses at first glance.

You can practice these poses as a sequence, or on their own if you are short on time and still looking for some relaxation time. These routines are great to do after a combination of the poses from the previous chapters as well.

Opposite Elbow Hold Reaching Up (Urdhva Hastasana Variation)

Body Areas Utilized: Arms, back, shoulders

Good For: Stretching the back and sides of the body and gaining mobility in the shoulders—although you are reaching up, which can often be energizing, the release from this pose will also provide you with relaxation and calming energy

Instructions

1. Sit up tall in the chair with your feet flat on the floor parallel to each other at hip-distance apart.

2. Gently and slowly raise both arms up toward the ceiling, bend your arms, and take hold of opposite elbows with your hands.

3. Look upward.

4. Hold here for an inhale then release your arms down as you exhale.

5. Repeat steps 2 through 4 eight to 10 times.

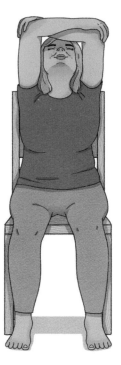

Tips

- Easier Variation: If you're having trouble holding the elbows or reaching straight up, keep the arms reaching out straight to the sides. You can also try holding one wrist, but remember to switch the grip to the other hand at some point to maintain the body's symmetry.

- Challenging Variation: Add a torso tilt each time you hold on to your elbows, alternating right to left.

Cautions

You might want to avoid practicing this pose if you are recovering from a back, neck, or shoulder injury, as it could cause strain in the muscles and joints of those areas.

Head Supported Arch

Body Areas Utilized: Arms, neck, shoulders, upper back

Good For: Increasing shoulder, upper back, and neck muscle flexibility and joint mobility, as well as stretching open the chest to prepare it for the more restful poses to follow

Instructions

1. Sit up tall in the chair with your feet flat on the floor parallel to each other at hip-distance apart.

2. Reach both arms out to the side and bend your elbows, placing your hands behind your head.

3. Slowly and gently arch your upper back, looking up slightly.

4. Hold here for three to five deep breaths.

5. Come out of the arch and release your hands and arms down.

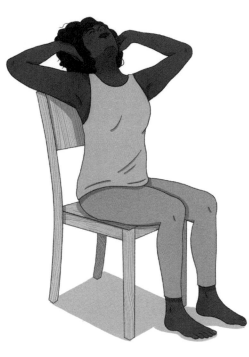

Tips

- Easier Variation: Leave out the upper-back arch and just complete the arm portion of the pose.

- Challenging Variation: Instead of placing your hands behind your head, reach your arms straight upward.

Cautions

You will want to skip this pose if you are recovering from a back, neck, shoulder, or arm injury. It requires you to support some of the weight of your head with your hands and arms, so if you have any sensitivity in the areas listed above and you choose to try this pose, please take care.

Wide-Legged Bend with Support

Body Areas Utilized: Arms, back, hamstrings, hips, inner thighs, neck

Good For: Stretching and gaining flexibility in the hips, inner thighs, and hamstrings, releasing tension from the back and neck muscles, and calming the mind and body

Instructions

1. Sit up tall in the chair and step your feet out as wide as you are able to go without strain or tension.

2. Place your hands on your thighs and slowly fold your torso over and down.

3. Keeping your hands on your legs for support, hold here for three to five deep breaths.

4. Use your hands to help you come up to an upright seated position.

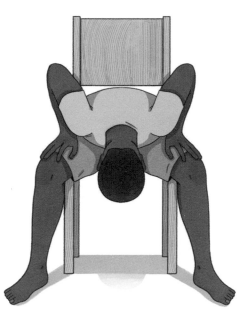

Tips

- Easier Variation: Keep your legs closer together and don't fold your torso over as far, keeping your head raised instead.

- Challenging Variation: Instead of keeping your hands on your thighs, place them flat on the ground or on a support, such as stacked yoga blocks.

Cautions

If you are recovering from a hip, back, neck, shoulder, or arm injury, you'll want to skip this pose. The weight of the head here, like with any forward-bending pose of this nature, can be a bit heavy for your neck to support. Please work with caution and come out of the pose if it causes any kind of neck pain.

Chair Half Lotus Pose (Chair Ardha Padmasana)

Body Areas Utilized: Hamstrings, hips, inner and outer thighs

Good For: Building hip flexibility and calming the mind and body by releasing tension in the hip joint

Instructions

1. Sit up tall on the chair with your feet flat on the floor parallel to each other at hip-distance apart.

2. Place your right ankle over your left thigh and bring your right knee out to the side.

3. Place your right hand on your right knee and your left hand on your right foot, keeping your hands relaxed and palms facing up.

4. Continue to sit up tall, close your eyes, and deepen your breath.

5. Breathe slowly and deeply through your nose, coming inward with your mind and focusing on your breath.

6. Remain here for 15 to 25 deep breaths.

7. When you are ready, slowly and gently come to open your eyes, release your hands, and uncross your leg.

8. Repeat steps 2 through 7 on the other side.

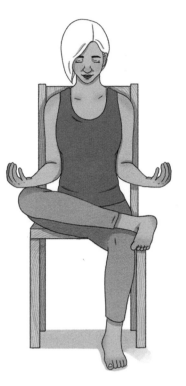

- Easier Variation: Instead of crossing your ankle over your thigh, just cross one thigh on top of the other and place your palms flat on your legs.

- Challenging Variation: Try this in a cross-legged position on the ground instead of sitting in the chair.

Cautions

You may want to avoid practicing this pose if you are recovering from a hip or leg injury. This is a deeper hip stretch, especially for the outer hip area, so please lessen the intensity of the stretch or come out of the pose if you feel any pain around the hip joint.

Supported Bound Angle Pose (Baddha Konasana)

Body Areas Utilized: Hamstrings, hips, inner thighs

Good For: A nice gentle stretch for the inner thighs and hips, quieting the mind and calming the body

Props Needed

One yoga bolster and two yoga blocks

Instructions

1. In front of the chair by your feet, place two yoga blocks at the medium height and place a yoga bolster flat on top of the yoga blocks so it is fully supported, keeping the structure on the ground.

2. Sit up tall in the chair and place your feet together in the center of your yoga bolster.

3. Bring your knees to rest, turning outward from the hips.

4. Place your hands on your thighs with your palms facing upward.

5. Sit up tall, close your eyes, and deepen your breath.

6. Breathe slowly and deeply through your nose, coming inward with your mind and focusing on your breath.

7. Remain here for 15 to 25 deep breaths.

8. When you are ready, open your eyes and release your hands and feet back to a neutral position.

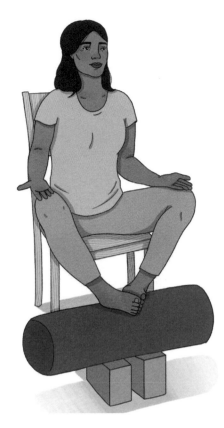

- Easier Variation: Try placing the yoga bolster structure slightly farther away from your chair so you can rest your feet on top of it with your legs out straight instead of keeping them in the bound angle position.

- Challenging Variation: Try doing the bound angle pose sitting on the ground with your feet together and knees relaxed out to the side.

Cautions

You may want to skip this pose if you are recovering from a hip injury. Because the weight of your legs is dropping outward due to gravity, the strain on your hips and inner thighs may be intense after a while, so please avoid or come out of this pose if you experience any pain in those areas.

10-Minute Sequence at a Glance

On these two pages, you will see images of all the poses described in your 10-minute Unwind and Sleep chair yoga routine at a glance so you can easily reference them while you practice.

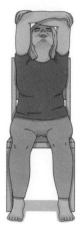

 Opposite Elbow Hold Reaching Up (Urdhva Hastasana Variation)
Hold for one deep breath. Perform eight to 10 times.

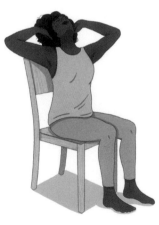

 Head Supported Arch
Hold for three to five breaths. Perform two to four times.

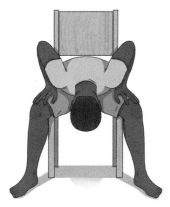

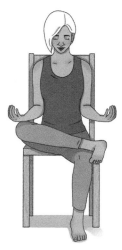

3 Wide-Legged Bend with Support
Hold for three to five breaths. Perform two to four times.

4 Chair Half Lotus Pose (Chair Ardha Padmasana)
Hold for 15 to 25 breaths on each side.

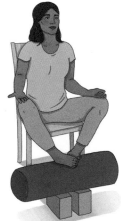

5 Supported Bound Angle Pose (Baddha Konasana)
Hold for 15 to 25 breaths.

Prayer Hands in Chair (Chair Anjali Mudra)

Body Areas Utilized: Arms, back

Good For: Calming the mind and grounding the body—it helps you center yourself and provides you with more focus

Instructions

1. Sit up tall in the chair with your feet flat on the floor, parallel at hip-distance apart.

2. Bring your hands to meet at the center of your chest and your elbows out to the side.

3. Close your eyes and deepen your breath.

4. Breathe deeply, coming inward with your mind and focusing on your breathing.

5. Remain here for 25 to 30 deep breaths.

6. When you are ready, slowly open your eyes.

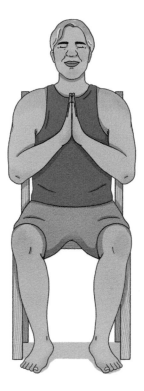

Tips

- Easier Variation: Keep your hands on your legs instead of in the prayer position.

- Challenging Variation: Try this meditation sitting in a cross-legged position either directly on the floor or on a support such as a folded blanket.

Cautions

You may want to skip this pose if you have trouble or discomfort while sitting down in the same position for long periods of time. This is a pose where you are able to practice meditation, which can be very helpful for healing, but if your body gets uncomfortable, you may want to find a more comfortable position.

Wide-Legged Side Bend

Body Areas Utilized: Arms, hips, inner thighs, sides of torso

Good For: Stretching and gaining flexibility in the hips, inner thighs, and sides of the torso—it's very lengthening for the side body, which will help provide more relaxation in the upcoming poses

Instructions

1. Sit up tall in the chair with your feet flat on the ground.

2. Bring your legs out to a wide position.

3. Place your left forearm on your left thigh and tilt your torso over to the left, reaching your right arm up and over on a diagonal.

4. Hold here for three to five deep breaths.

5. Slowly and gently lift your torso back upright and remove your arm from your leg.

6. Repeat steps 3 through 5 on the other side.

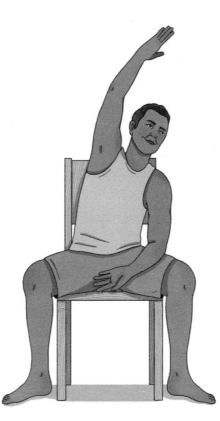

Tips

- Easier Variation: Keep both your hands on both thighs and gently tilt your torso to the side.

- Challenging Variation: Try bringing your legs out wider and bending your raised arm, bringing your hand behind your back for a deeper shoulder and chest opening stretch.

Cautions

You may want to skip this pose if you are recovering from a side, back, hip, or arm injury. The stretching of the sides of the torso can be quite deep for someone who is recovering from an injury or is sensitive in that area. If you choose to practice this, you can lessen the intensity of the stretch or come out of the pose sooner than instructed.

Hands Over Heart in Chair

. . . .

Body Areas Utilized: Arms, back

Good For: Calming the mind and grounding the body by helping you focus your attention within

. . . .

Instructions

1. Sit up tall in the chair with your feet flat and parallel on the floor at hip-distance apart.

2. Bring your hands to your chest, placing one on top of the other over your heart's center.

3. Close your eyes and deepen your breath.

4. Breathe deeply, coming inward with your mind and focusing on your breathing.

5. Remain here for 25 to 30 deep breaths.

6. When you are ready, slowly open your eyes.

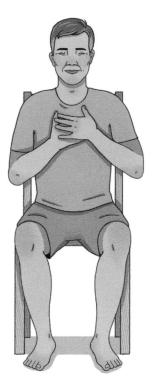

Tips

- Easier Variation: Keep your hands on your legs instead of over your heart.

- Challenging Variation: Try this meditation sitting in a cross-legged position either directly on the floor or on a support such as a folded blanket.

Cautions

You may want to skip this pose if you have trouble or discomfort while sitting down in the same position for long periods of time. This is another meditative pose, so if you are uncomfortable, you may want to find a new position.

Hand to Heart and Hand to Belly in a Chair

Body Areas Utilized: Arms, back

Good For: Calming the mind and grounding the body—you'll be able to feel your breath in a different way and connect more deeply with your body

Instructions

1. Sit up tall in the chair with your feet flat and parallel on the floor at hip-distance apart.

2. Bring one hand to your heart's center and the other to your belly.

3. Close your eyes and deepen your breath.

4. Breathe deeply, coming inward with your mind and focusing on your breathing.

5. Remain here for 25 to 30 deep breaths.

6. When you are ready, slowly open your eyes.

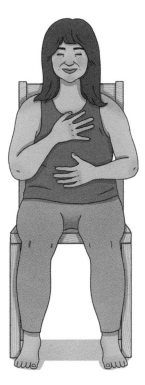

Tips

- Easier Variation: Keep your hands on your legs instead of on your heart and belly.

- Challenging Variation: Try this meditation sitting in a cross-legged position either directly on the floor or on a support such as a folded blanket.

Cautions

You may want to skip this pose if you have trouble or discomfort while sitting down in the same position for long periods of time. Or, as mentioned earlier, try to find a different position, perhaps lying down on a bed or comfortable surface, to practice this meditation.

Two-Chair Supported Rest

Body Areas Utilized: Back, hips

Good For: Calming the mind and body to relax and unwind

Props Needed

One extra chair and a yoga bolster

Instructions

1. Place the extra chair in front of you with a yoga bolster resting on both chairs, creating a bridge between the two.

2. Be sure that the bolster is stable, then rest your entire torso on top of the bolster with one arm on either side of it.

3. Turn your head to the left, resting your right cheek on the bolster.

4. Close your eyes and deepen your breath.

5. Turn your mind inward, focusing on your inhales and exhales.

6. Remain here for 15 to 20 deep breaths.

7. Gently lift your head up and turn it to the opposite side, resting it back down on the bolster.

8. Repeat steps 4 through 7.

9. Slowly open your eyes, then lift your head and torso to an upright seated position.

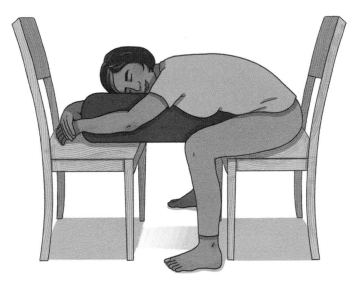

Tips

- Easier Variation: Substitute this pose with the Prayer Hands pose (page 110), the Hands Over Heart pose (page 114), or the Hand to Heart and Hand to Belly pose (page 116).

- Challenging Variation: Try this pose sitting on the ground in a cross-legged or straight-legged position with the torso resting on one or several stacked bolsters, depending on your flexibility.

Cautions

You may want to skip this pose if you are recovering from a back, hip, or neck injury, or if you have trouble sitting in one place for long periods of time. When using your bolster to create a bridge, make sure the chairs are close enough together that the bolster doesn't sag or fall between them.

Seated Forward Bend on a Chair

....

Body Areas Utilized: Arms, back, hips, shoulders

Good For: Calming the mind and body to relax and unwind

....

Props Needed

Two yoga blankets

Instructions

1. Sit on the ground on top of a folded yoga blanket, facing the seat of the chair.

2. Have the second folded yoga blanket on top of the seat of the chair.

3. Cross your shins, flex your feet under your knees, and sit up tall with your spine straight.

4. When you are ready, fold your torso forward, bend your arms, and stack your hands one on top of the other in front of you on the seat of the chair.

5. Place your forehead on top of your hands and rest there in a forward bend.

6. Close your eyes and deepen your breathing.

7. Quiet your mind by coming inward and focusing on your inhales and exhales.

8. Remain here for 25 to 30 deep breaths.

9. When you are ready, slowly come back to an upright seated position and open your eyes.

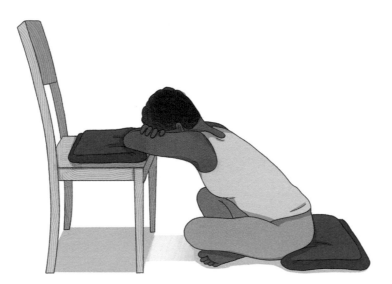

Tips

- Easier Variation: Instead of folding forward, you can sit up tall in a cross-legged position on the ground and remain there.

- Challenging Variation: Instead of crossing your legs, you can keep them straight on either side of the chair in front of you.

Cautions

You may want to skip this pose if you are recovering from a hip, leg, neck, shoulder, or back injury. Otherwise, be gentle when leaning forward, because the stretching can be more intense than you might expect.

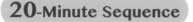

Legs on a Chair (Savasana Variation)

Body Areas Utilized: Back, hips, legs

Good For: Calming the mind and body to relax and unwind

Instructions

1. Lie flat on the ground with your hips facing the front of the chair.

2. Bring your hips close enough to the chair that you can rest your calves on the seat.

3. Bring both legs to the seat of the chair and keep them at hip-distance apart.

4. Bring your hands down by your sides on the ground with your palms facing up.

5. Close your eyes and deepen your breathing.

6. Quiet your mind by coming inward and focusing on your inhales and exhales.

7. Remain here for 25 to 30 deep breaths.

8. When you are ready, gently remove your legs from the chair and come back to an upright seated position, then open your eyes.

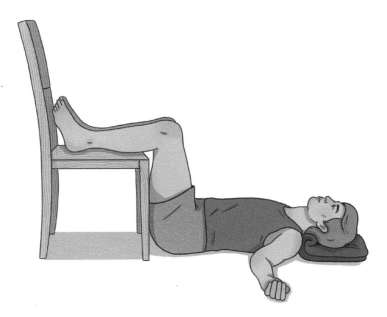

Tips

- Easier Variation: Try lying flat on the ground with a rolled-up blanket under your knees for lower-back support.

- Challenging Variation: Rest your legs on a wall, keeping them straight, for a slightly deeper leg stretch.

Cautions

You may want to skip this pose if you are recovering from a back, hip, or leg injury, or if you have trouble lying in one spot for long periods of time. In that case, find a more comfortable position to meditate in for this amount of time or try one of the earlier seated poses.

20-Minute Sequence at a Glance

On these two pages, you will see images of all the poses described in your 20-minute Unwind and Sleep chair yoga routine at a glance so you can easily reference them while you practice.

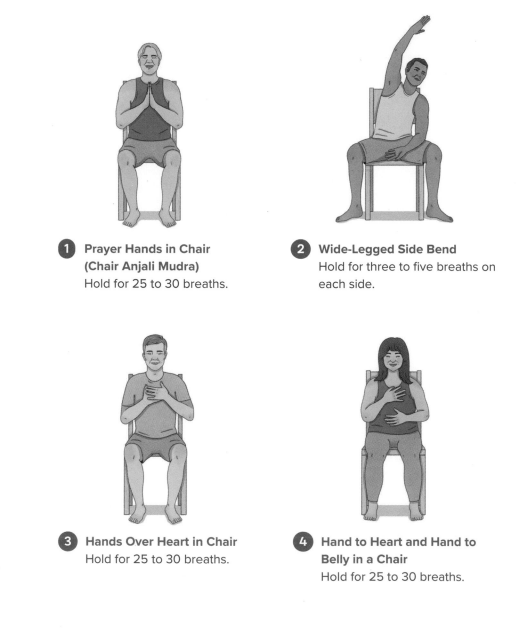

1 **Prayer Hands in Chair (Chair Anjali Mudra)**
Hold for 25 to 30 breaths.

2 **Wide-Legged Side Bend**
Hold for three to five breaths on each side.

3 **Hands Over Heart in Chair**
Hold for 25 to 30 breaths.

4 **Hand to Heart and Hand to Belly in a Chair**
Hold for 25 to 30 breaths.

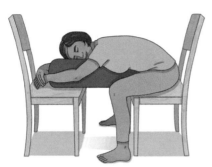

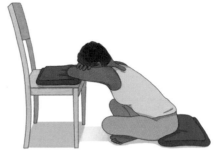

 Two-Chair Supported Rest
Hold for 15 to 20 breaths on each side.

6 **Seated Forward Bend on a Chair**
Hold for 25 to 30 breaths.

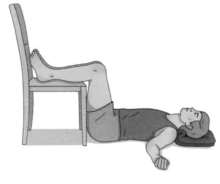

 Legs on a Chair (Savasana Variation)
Hold for 25 to 30 breaths.

Still the Mind with Yogic Breathwork

In the yogic tradition, there are several types of breathing techniques that are incorporated into a yoga practice along with physical and mental exercises. This yogic breathing technique is referred to as *pranayama,* which means "drawing out the lifeforce." Pranayama is one of the eight limbs of yoga—the ancient yogic guidelines on how to live a meaningful and purposeful life. In the yoga philosophy, breathing techniques and breathwork are very important to the overall process.

The following breathing techniques can be very simple to try and they help soothe the body and calm the mind.

Breath Awareness

Practice When: You are sitting quietly in meditation or in a restorative yoga pose

Instructions

1. Sit up tall in a chair or on the ground, or lie down with your spine straight.
2. Close your eyes and breathe deeply through your nose.
3. Bring your awareness to your breathing, noticing each inhale and exhale, and keep your attention there.
4. You can count your breath, notice the pathway of your breath as it travels in and out of your body, or notice how your body feels with each inhale and exhale.
5. Breathe at a normal and natural pace and keep your attention there for as long as you would like to.

Victorious Breath (Ujjayi Breath)

Practice When: You are doing the physical postures of yoga and/or looking to build heat and warmth in your body.

Instructions

1. You can do this while seated, but once you get comfortable with this breath, you can do it during your physical yoga asana practice.

2. Breathe in through your nose and out through your mouth with a "hah" sound, as if you are fogging up a mirror. It can also be helpful to put your hand up to your mouth as you are breathing out to feel the steam on your palm.

3. Repeat that several times until you feel comfortable doing so.

4. Once you are ready, try completing the exhale with your mouth closed while still being able to hear your exhale and getting that feeling of the breath in the back of your throat.

5. Your breath should be audible enough that someone right next to you can hear you, but not any further than that.

6. Repeat this for as many times as needed to build heat and warmth in your body.

Alternate Nostril Breathing (Nadi Shodhana)

Practice When: You want to calm down the mind and body and cultivate mental focus. This is not appropriate for anyone who shouldn't be practicing breath retention (that is, if you are pregnant or have blocked sinuses, cold/flu, or fever).

Instructions

1. Find a comfortable position sitting up tall with your spine straight.
2. Place your left hand on your thigh and fold the fingers of your right hand so that only your pinky finger and your thumb are out.
3. Place your thumb on your right nostril, blocking the airway, and inhale deeply through your left nostril.
4. Hold the breath, place your pinky finger on the left nostril, and release the thumb from the right nostril to exhale.
5. Inhale through the right nostril, hold the breath, and place the thumb back on the right nostril while releasing the pinky finger from the left to exhale.
6. Continue with this breath pattern for three to five breaths, release the hand, and return to your normal breathing.

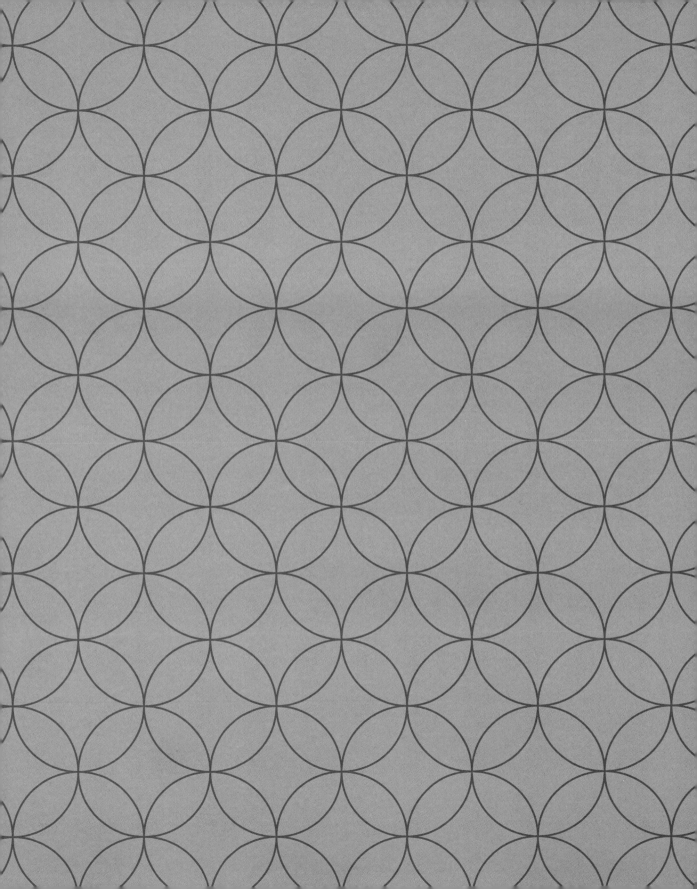

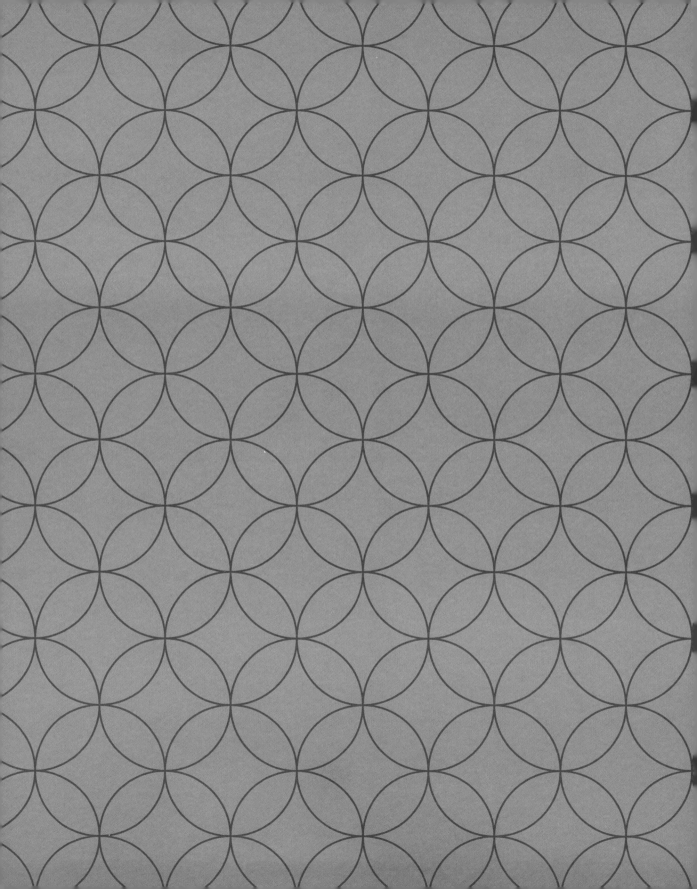

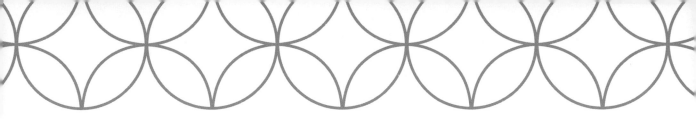

RESOURCES AND REFERENCES

Print Books

Iyengar, B. K. S. *Light on Yoga*. Revised ed. New York: Schocken Books, 1979.

Farhi, Donna. *Yoga Mind, Body & Spirit: A Return to Wholeness*. New York: Henry Holt and Company, 2000.

Websites

VeryWellFit.com

HealthLine.com

YogaJournal.com

DoYou.com

ChriskaYoga.com

YouTube.com/c/ChriskaYoga

INDEX

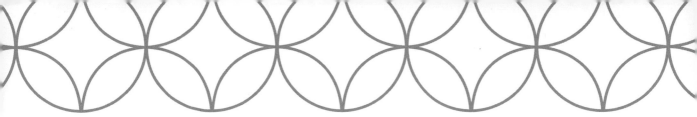

ACKNOWLEDGMENTS

I would like to thank all those at Callisto Media for providing me with another opportunity to share my knowledge of yoga with a wider audience. I would also like to thank my editor, Eun H. Jeong, for guiding the writing process along and being so patient and helpful.

I would like to thank my parents, Lisa and Joe, for always being there for me and for their constant lifetime of support.

A huge thank you to my husband, Barry, for his love and support throughout the process of writing this book and beyond.

Last but not least, I would like to thank all the supporters of my Yoga With Christina YouTube channel. Their incredible kindness and constant support are what keeps me motivated to continue sharing the message of yoga with the world.

ABOUT THE AUTHOR

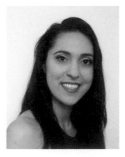

Christina D'Arrigo is a 500-hour-trained yoga teacher and former dancer/choreographer from New York City. As a former attendee of the *Fame* school in New York City, Christina received her specialized high school diploma in dance and then went on to study dance in Los Angeles and London, where she received her bachelor's and master's degrees in dance and choreography. Upon her return to New York City, she completed her 500-hour yoga teacher training and began teaching yoga classes live and online for thousands of people all over the world via the YouTube channel Yoga With Christina–ChriskaYoga and various other platforms.